I0711252

# STOP OVEREATING

*Guide to Overcome Emotional and Binge Eating, End to Eat in Compulsive Way, Lose Excess Weight Approaching a Mindful and Intuitive Eating.*

## By

## LINDA CRUMP

© Copyright 2020 By LINDA CRUMP

All rights reserved.

This document is geared towards providing exact and reliable information with regards to the topic and issue covered. The publication is sold with the idea that the publisher is not required to render accounting, officially permitted, or otherwise, qualified services. If advice is necessary, legal or professional, a practiced individual in the profession should be ordered.

From a Declaration of Principles which was accepted and approved equally by a Committee of the American Bar Association and a Committee of Publishers and Associations.

In no way is it legal to reproduce, duplicate, or transmit any part of this document in either electronic means or in printed format. Recording of this publication is strictly prohibited and any storage of this document is not allowed unless with written permission from the publisher. All rights reserved.

The information provided herein is stated to be truthful and consistent, in that any liability, in terms of inattention or otherwise, by any usage or abuse of any policies, processes, or directions contained within is the solitary and utter responsibility of the recipient reader. Under no circumstances will any legal responsibility or blame be held against the publisher for any reparation, damages, or monetary loss due to the information herein, either directly or indirectly.

Respective authors own all copyrights not held by the publisher.

The information herein is offered for informational purposes solely, and is universal as so. The presentation of the information is without contract or any type of guarantee assurance.

The trademarks that are used are without any consent, and the publication of the trademark is without permission or backing by the trademark owner. All trademarks and brands within this book are for clarifying purposes only and are the owned by the owners themselves, not affiliated with this document.

# Table of Content


INTRODUCTION ..................................................... 1

**CHAPTER ONE:** WHAT IS OVEREATING .............. 3

HOW TO STOP OVEREATING ...................... 8

WHAT KIND OF EATER ARE YOU? ..................... 14

**CHAPTER TWO:** EMOTIONAL EATING .............. 19

WHY CANT I MANAGE MY EMOTIONS?.......... 53

COMPULSIVE EATING ........................... 59

**CHAPTER THREE:** BINGE EATING...................... 69

**CHAPTER FOUR:** QUIT FOCUSSING ON WEIGHT LOSS FOCUS ON HEALTH INSTEAD ................... 107

THE PRACTICE OF MINFUL EATING .............. 118

BODY SENSATION AND MINFUL RELATIONSHIP WITH FOOD ........................... 144

**CHAPTER FIVE:** DEALING WITH YOUR EMOTIONS ............................................... 153

# INTRODUCTION

Nourishment and weight issues and related self-perception issues influence an enormous part of the total populace. You might be one of the over 1.4 billion grown-ups over the world (in 2008) who were overweight and the greater part a billion who were viewed as corpulent (World Health Organization 2014). Regardless of whether you aren't overweight or large, you may battle with nourishment issues, for example, nourishment desires, nourishment fears, or habitual overeating. You may additionally have self-perception issues in which you feel your body has double-crossed you by not being the size or shape you'd need it to be, or out of the blue, you may feel disappointed with your body. On the off chance that any of that is valid, you might be investing a ton of your energy agonizing over your appearance or body size, attempting to get in shape or battling not to recover weight you've lost, attempting counts calories, stressing over looking for garments, and feeling embarrassed about what you look like. By presently, you may have additionally understood that eating less junk food doesn't work—in any event not over the long haul. In the event that you are feeling miserable or you feel as though nothing has truly worked for you, at that point this book will bode well.

This book is structured in a way to help you overcome overeating issues which may stem from any of:

- Emotional eating
- Compulsive eating, and
- Binge eating

This book will assist you with understanding why you've experienced such difficulty with your weight. You will figure out how your weight, nourishment, and self-perception issues are associated with encounters you may have had as a youngster or grown-up, to your feelings, and to convictions you've shaped (normally unwittingly) about yourself and life that keep you stuck. Yet, other than letting you know the "why" of your nourishment and weight issues, this book will furnish you with approaches to evacuate these squares and furthermore handy and feasible answers for the normal entanglements that a great many people with nourishment, weight, and self-perception issues battle with—issues, for example, how to stop emotional eating, manage worry without nourishment, and expel squares to moving your body.

# CHAPTER ONE
## *WHAT IS OVEREATING*

Gorging is a typical issue. It can prompt different issues, running from indigestion in the short term to heftiness in the long haul. It has additionally been seen as related to many GImanifestations, including stomach torment, especially in the upper gastrointestinal tract, swelling, and looseness of the bowels. Eating an excess of one time won't cause heftiness; however, it might cause distress, torment, and impedance with rest.

Even though we may expect that these side effects would demoralize individuals from gorging, shockingly, the body acclimates to indulging by discharging dopamine. This natural joy substance urges us to eat even more. So regardless of whether indulging causes torment and distress, we may feel constrained to keep gorging. This is a significant piece of how nourishment habit creates. So over a more drawn out timeframe, gorging all the time, without sufficient exercise, can prompt weight.

At the point when we eat nourishments we appreciate, the body discharges dopamine, which is related to sentiments of delight or prize, and it urges us to eat significantly more. So regardless of whether indulging causes agony and inconvenience, we may feel constrained to keep gorging. What's more, just to make the circumstance significantly progressively confounded, there isn't only one sort of gorging. It can occur as a consequence of how you feel, who you are with, and numerous different elements. Here are ten of the most now and again referred to kinds of indulging that can prompt torment and corpulence, as can add to the advancement of nourishment enslavement.

Here are ten of the most as often as possible referred to ways that indulging can turn into an issue. Envision your preferred nourishments for a moment: pizza, french fries, steak, potato chips. Simply contemplating them likely makes you eager, isn't that so? Past furnishing us with the vitality we have to live, nourishment can be a significant wellspring of joy. It tastes great and has numerous fragrances, surfaces, and different highlights that allure the faculties. For a few, nourishment is likewise a passionate adapting device. You may gorge when you're feeling pushed, pitiful, or stressed. Lamentably, gorging (even your preferred nourishments) can damage your wellbeing.

Here's a glance at why you're likely indulging and how to be more careful at eating times. Recall the last time you ate so much you felt utterly stuffed. Were you attacking an immense cake to praise a companion's birthday? Stacking up on turkey and sweet potatoes at Thanksgiving? Or then again, were you at home alone, perhaps toward the finish of an extreme day? How could you feel subsequently - basically irritated that you gave yourself a stomach-ache? Or, on the other hand were you tormented by blame or disgrace?

Eating a lot of now and again is typical. So is eating for passionate reasons. "From the minute we're conceived, we're sustained with nourishment, remunerated with nourishment; thus, enthusiastic associations with nourishment are typical," says Michelle May, MD, creator of Eat What You Love, Love What You Eat. of adapting to negative feelings. As a result, they frequently feel that their eating is wild. They consider nourishment always and feel remorseful, embarrassed, or on the other hand, discouraged after eating. "That is unique in relation to what somebody feels after, state, eating a major Thanksgiving dinner," May says. "You may feel full; also, you may lament having had that last cut of pie, yet you're most certainly not overwhelmed by disgrace."

**Why you're indulging**

Have you at any point asked why you go after nourishment when you're feeling a compelling feeling? You're not the only one. Numerous components shape dietary patterns, including anything from social standards to monetary status to mental issues. Numerous individuals eat when they are attempting to adapt to emotions.

Eating may at first seem like assistance to ease pressure or uneasiness. Sooner or later, however, with self-perception issues, prompting a pattern of — yes — increasingly enthusiastic eating. A few people who gorge have a clinical turmoil called voraciously consuming food clutter (BED). Individuals with BED impulsively eat a lot of nourishment in a short measure of time and feel blame or disgrace a while later. Furthermore, you probably won't do it consistently, however, just when you're feeling pushed, forlorn, or upset.

**How can it start?**

Now and again, individuals essentially gorge out of careless propensity, as usual plunking down with a sack of chips in front of the TV around evening time. Be that as it may, in many cases, it's the aftereffect of fundamental enthusiastic issues. Having a negative body picture can assume a significant job. For some individuals, urgent indulging is a piece of a cycle that begins with a prohibitive eating routine. May considers it the "eat, atone, rehash" cycle. You may start an eating routine since you feel awful about your weight or size yet find that it's too difficult to even think about sticking to - mainly if you use nourishment as an adapting instrument.

In the long run, you hit a limit furthermore, gorge on "illegal" nourishments, and at that point, the blame and disgrace set in, and the limitations start once more. The cycle can be challenging to break. "Indeedindividuals who state they're not on a tight eating routine regularly have instilled thoughts regarding 'great' or 'awful' nourishments," says Marsha Hudnall, leader of Green Mountain at Fox Run in Vermont, an inside for ladies who battle with gorging. "In any case, when you have a substance that is normally engaging and mitigating and soothing, and you make it beyond reach, it just turns out to be progressively appealing."

Passionate eating may even prompt a progressively genuine condition like gorge dietary issues (BED). This issue includes eating a lot of nourishment exceptionally. You may feel wild during a voraciously consuming food scene and unfit to stop. It might feel like a solid impulse. A few people gorge on exceptional occasions, similar to occasions or birthday celebrations. With BED, gorging may begin to happen all the more as often as possible and with no event by any means. You may feel humiliated about your dietary patterns and attempt over and over to stop.

Different indications of BED include:

- eating until you're awkwardly full
- eating stealthily
- eating a lot of nourishment in a set measure of time, similar to an hour visit eating fewer carbs with or without weight-reduction BED is extremely hard to defeat all alone. It might prompt heftiness and related illnesses like sort 2 diabetes, coronary disease, and gastroesophageal reflux illness become a famous thought among a few researchers.

Those analysts state that certain nourishments high in fat, sugar, and salt are addictive, causing changes in the mind like those made by drugs. Studies in creatures have indicated that rodents that gorge on sugar, for instance, can create indications of reliance.

Be that as it may, the possibility of nourishment dependence is questionable. For a specific something, the standard treatment for fixation is restraint, and that is impractical with nourishment. Likewise, "eating less junk food is a substantial segment of the voraciously consuming food cycle," May says. "From that angle, it's counterproductive to mark certain nourishments as negative."

There's no uncertainty that eating can animate the arrival of feel-better synthetic substances in mind, Hudnall says. "In any case, that doesn't make nourishment an addictive substance. There's proof that it's the conduct — the limit/gorge cycle - that causes the indications of reliance, not the nourishment itself," she says. A few analysts have even expressed that the expression "eating fixation" is an increasingly exact term than "nourishment fixation."

## HOW TO STOP OVEREATING

Look for help. It very well may be difficult to stop gorging all alone, especially if there are profound established enthusiastic issues included, says Robin B. Kanarek, PhD, teacher of brain science mental triggers - like a negative self-perception - that might be driving your conduct.

Stay away from marks. "Comprehend that you're not a terrible individual doing awful things," May says.

"Naming yourself can become an inevitable outcome in terms of proceeding with the cycle."

The equivalent goes for naming nourishments. "Nourishment is nourishment - it's 'bad' or 'awful,'"

Kanarek says. "It tends to be difficult to get over those profoundly held convictions, yet inquire about shows that on the off chance that you eat what you consider a 'terrible' nourishment, you're more prone to indulge a short time later."

Take a respite. At the point when you feel like eating, briefly stop and inquire yourself: Am I hungry? "Once in a while individuals get so centered around what they need to eat that they don't stop and wonder why they need to eat,"

May says. If you use nourishment as an adapting instrument, you might be withdrawn from the prompts that sign appetite or totality, and it's essential to bring your mindfulness back to your body.

Change your condition. "A propensity is all the time conduct that is on autopilot," Hudnall says. Making a change to your condition can return your concentration to your conduct and allow you to make a more intentional choice. For instance,

Hudnall says, "on the off chance that you generally sit in a certain seat to eat, move it to an elsewhere altogether." Surrender to desires - with some restraint. Forbidding nourishments can make you gorge them later on. In case you truly need something - regardless of whether you're most certainly not hungry - authorize yourself to have a modest quantity.

End prohibitive weight control plans. "Gorging and prohibitive eating are regularly different sides of a similar coin," May says. "Hardship can be a trigger for gorging simply like stress, outrage, or tension."

1. Distinguish your triggers

You may initially need to keep a nourishment journal so you can write down how you're feeling when you're gorging. Is it accurate to say that you are tragic, restless, or exhausted? Compose it down. Do you will, in general, snatch specific nourishment when you're gorging? Make notes on that also. When you begin to see an example, you can chip away at supplanting gorging with more advantageous methods for dealing with stress.

2. Eat all the more gradually

On the off chance that you, despite everything, feel like you have to eat, take a stab at making it gradually. Your stomach, in reality, takes around 20 minutes to speak with your cerebrum that you are full of eating. Thus, bite every significant piece a few times. Set aside an effort to appreciate the flavors and surfaces in your supper. When you've completed a dinner or, on the other hand nibble, enjoy a reprieve to check whether you're full before eating more.

3. Try not to skip dinners

In case you're particularly eager, you might be bound to the gorge. Numerous individuals skip breakfast, yet eating promptly in the day may support you keep up a substantial weight and oppose gorging. Truth be told, having breakfast may build the dopamine levels in your cerebrum. Dopamine has the force to help control longings and your motivation to gorge.

4. Eat entire nourishments

Going after more advantageous nourishments may ease gorging. At the point when you eat prepared nourishments, especially straightforward starches, or different food sources high in sugar, your glucose spikes and later crashes. Subsequently, you become covetously ravenous once more. Prepared nourishments incorporate anything from candy bars to sugary breakfast oat to pasta made with white flour.

What would it be a good idea for you to eat? Have a go at staying with entire nourishments, for example, vegetables, organic products, nuts, whole grains (complex starches), fish, grass-fed meats, and solid fats like olive oil.

5. Get great rest

At the point when you're drained, you may eat more than expected. An ongoing report shows that poor rest is legitimately identified with both expanded pressure and passionate eating in ladies. The ladies were given snacks in a research center and put under upsetting conditions. The individuals who had rested soundly didn't eat so much as the individuals who hadn't had enough closed eye. Point to get somewhere in the range of seven and eight hours of rest every night.

6. Accomplish something different

Inclining that you can't control yourself? Avoid the washroom. Attempt supplanting your gorging with another movement. Exercise is an incredible alternative that may even assist with improving your self-perception. You might need to take a stroll around the square, go running, or head to the exercise center to lift a few loads. Besides work out, there are numerous different approaches to control pressure.

In case you're despite everything feeling crazy, you don't need to battle alone. It might be a smart thought to contact your primary care physician, particularly if you feel that you may be creating BED. You may profit by intellectual conduct treatment (CBT). This sort of treatment causes you to perceive designs by the way you consider nourishment.

In treatment, you may chip away at positive adapting abilities, including self-statements. For instance, you may feel vanquished and think: "Halting gorging is excessively hard, I can't do it." In CBT, you would work to perceive this thought and react to it by saying to yourself: "I understand right now that I am indulging. I presently should consider how I can quit surrendering to this conduct."

There are a lot more things you can do to quit gorging. You can begin changing your propensities when you go to take your next chomp of nourishment. Here are some more tips for rehearsing careful, proper dieting:

When to see your PCP

In case you're despite everything feeling crazy, you don't need to battle alone. It might be a smart thought to contact your PCP, mainly if you think that you may be creating BED. You may profit by psychological conduct treatment (CBT). This kind of treatment causes you to perceive designs by the way you consider nourishment.

In treatment, you may take a shot at positive adapting aptitudes, including self-statements. For instance, you may feel crushed and think: "Halting gorging is excessively hard, I can't do it." In CBT, you would work to perceive this thought and react to it by saying to yourself: "I understand right now that I am indulging. I currently should consider how I can quit yielding to this conduct." There are prescriptions you can take for BED. These incorporate antidepressants (particular serotonin reuptake inhibitors or SSRIs) and Topamax (topiramate), an anticonvulsant that may diminish gorging scenes. A few people likewise advantage from conduct weight reduction programs.

# WHAT KIND OF EATER ARE YOU?

1.  Voracious Eater

    Voraciously consuming food includes expending a lot of nourishment in a short space of time. Gorges, by de€ nition, require you to eat more nourishment than individuals typically do, and more nourishment than you need. Voraciously consuming food can occur in an isolated event, or it can turn into a common method for eating, prompting issues.

Although voraciously consuming food in itself doesn't establish nourishment enslavement or dietary problem, overeatingis a side effect of Binge Eating Disorder and the dietary issue Bulimia Nervosa.

2.  Indulging From Supersize Meal Portions

Supersize supper parcels are normally the extra-enormous bits of cheap food or café feast servings, whereby the nourishment partition you purchase is a lot bigger than a typical feast divide. Supersize feast divides are intensely advertised, especially in North American culture. This can undoubtedly prompt expending a lot bigger measures of nourishment than would normally be appropriate and, whenever eaten all the time, can prompt corpulence and poor sustenance.

3.  Emotional Eater

Regularly referred to on shows, for example, Oprah, emotional eating is often alluded to as a way that ladies, in specific, eat when they feel resentful or miserable. The buzzwords of the young lady eating a quart of frozen yogurt after a terrible separation, or the moderately aged ladies gorging on carbs when she has PMS, are instances of "enthusiastic eating" generalizations.

Tragically these generalizations can prompt the very conduct they depict in individuals who identify with them. What's more, men experience enthusiastic eating too. One we would all be able to identify with. Regardless of whether it's a significant separation, an awful day busy working, or you viewed Forrest Gump once more; we've all gone to nourishment amid themisery. This kind of eater is probably going to be discovered wailing into a tub of dessert, takeaway eateries on speed dial, encompassed by void sweet wrappers. Can't thump this sort of eater an excessive amount of because it's happened to us all. Typically brings about a perpetual winding of disgrace as you get logically progressively resentful about the measure of nourishment you have quite recently eaten. If you know an Emotional Eater, give them an embrace.

4.  Stress Eating

Stress eating, albeit firmly identified with emotional eating, is more vigorously determined by nervousness as opposed to the gloom, and might be a method for energizing workaholic behavior when the time isn't taken for satisfactory breaks or suppers.

## 5.  The Healthy Eater

The kind of eater we should all try to be, aside from without the braggadocious holier-than-thou mentality. Indeed, we get that you're overly substantial. No, we would prefer not to think about it. These are the individuals who find a good pace to crush spirulina, honey bee dust and matcha smoothie before their everyday morning run. They come into work with their serving of mixed greens bowl also, reveal to you how much sugar is in the natural product juice you're drinking while causing to notice what number of various superfoods they have in their lunch. On the off chance that eating that solid makes you that horrendous, we'll adhere to the burgers, much appreciated.

## 6.  Sugar Addiction

Sweet, sugary nourishment is uniquely addictive to numerous individuals. Some overeaters gorge on confectionary or other sweet nourishments, with chocolate having a specific appeal. Guardians ought to be cautious that their kids don't create sugar compulsion, as everyday desserts utilization in adolescence is identified with passionate difficulties in adulthood, just as weight and tooth rot.

7.  Impulsive Snacking

Although eating a few snacks per day between dinners are frequently viewed as reliable, steady nibbling, especially on unfortunate tidbits, can prompt gorging, regardless of whether the eating is instead of or notwithstanding ordinary suppers. Many overeaters fall into the snare of cautiously arranging three solid suppers daily; however, not remembering snacks for their carbohydrate content, along these lines unintentionally gorging. The Midnight Snacker is pulled in to the gleam of the cooler like a moth to a flame. They'll be lying in bed, stomach protesting, and they'll hear the dessert in the cooler getting out their name. They'll roll out the familiar proverb that you ought to never rest hungry and creep down the stairs under the front of dimness to satiate their yearning. Nothing is sheltered from the Midnight Snacker. Is it safe to say that you were sparing those scraps for work tomorrow? Anticipating eating that cake in the cooler? No more.

8.  Inexpensive Food

Individuals who depend on inexpensive food regularly indulge. Cheap food is intended to animate indulging, normally by utilizing a mix of sugar, salt, and fat, all demonstrated by research to be addictive. Despite the fact that the elements of inexpensive food might be low quality and unappetizing, the addictive fixings guarantee a gigantic turnover of fatty nourishment, which can prompt corpulence and poor sustenance.

## 9.  Solace Eating

While comfort eating can be sound with some restraint, individuals who eat so as to manage troubling feelings may indulge and, likewise to pressure eaters and enthusiastic eaters, comfort eaters, may fall into the snare of nourishment addiction as their essential adapting methodology.

## 10. Social Eating

Social eating is a generally acknowledged practice and, with some restraint, can be a robust action. In any case, individuals who are continually compelled to eat socially, for example, the individuals who routinely go out on the town others, or individuals who meet over business dinners, might be inclined to gorging, especially when the desire is for enormous segments and unhealthy nourishments.

## 11. Fatigue Eating

Fatigue eating is a thoughtless way to deal with nourishment, in which an absence of incitement in different everyday issues prompts eating, just to feel something. Fatigue eaters can be inclined to gorging, supersize divides, urgent nibbling, sugar fixation, and cheap food.

# CHAPTER TWO
## *EMOTIONAL EATING*

### What is emotional eating?

Emotional eating is the inclination of its sufferers to react to unpleasant, delicate sentiments by eating, in any event, when not encountering physical hunger. Emotional eating or emotional appetite is frequently a desire for unhealthy or high-sugar nourishments that have insignificant dietary esteem. The nourishments that emotional eaters desire iscommonly alluded to as solace food sources, similar to dessert, treats, chocolate, chips, French fries, what's more, pizza. About 40% of individuals will in general eat more when focused, while about 40% eat less, and 20% experience no adjustment in the measure of nourishment they eat when presented to pressure. Subsequently, stress can be related with both weight put on and weight reduction. While emotional eating can be a side effect of what psychological well-being experts call atypical gloom, numerous individuals who don't have clinical discouragement or some other psychological well-being issue participate right now reaction to flitting sentiments or ceaseless pressure. This conduct is profoundly normal and is signi|cant since it can meddle with keeping up a sound eating regimen and add to weight.

### Emotional eating realities

Emotional eating is reacting to sentiments, for example, worry by eating high-sugar, fatty nourishments with low wholesome esteem. The amount of nourishment that is devoured is the essential contrast between emotional eating and pigging out. Like most emotional side effects, emotional eating is thought to result from various factors instead of a solitary reason. There are various potential admonition finishes paperwork for emotional eating, or stress eating. Wellbeing experts evaluate emotional eating by screening for physical and psychological wellness issues.

Conquering emotional eating includes showing the individual more beneficial approaches to see nourishment and grow better eating propensities (for example, careful eating), perceive their triggers for taking part right now, create other progressively suitable approaches to forestall and reduce pressure. At the point when untreated, emotional overeating can mess heftiness, up with weight reduction, and even lead to nourishment habit. Decreasing pressure, utilizing nourishment as sustenance as opposed to as an approach to take care of issues, and utilizing valuable approaches to deal with feelings can assist with forestalling emotional eating.

**What is the distinction between emotional eating and gorging?**

The essential distinction between emotional eating and voraciously consuming food includes the measure of nourishment that is expended. While both may include a feeling of difficulty controlling a hankering for nourishment, emotional eating may include expending from moderate to incredible measures of nourishment and may be the main manifestation that an individual has or be a piece of an emotional ailment like misery, bulimia, or voraciously consuming food issue. Voraciously consuming food scatter is an unmistakable psychological sickness that is portrayed by repetitive scenes of impulsive overeating, in that influenced individuals wildly eat a measure of nourishment that is significantly bigger than that which a great many people eat in an unmistakable timeframe (for instance, more than two hours), in any event, when they are not ravenous. The individual with pigging out turmoil may eat every a lot quicker than typical, hide the sum they eat out of disgrace, and may feel disturbed by their eating subsequent to doing as such. So as to fit the bill for this conclusion, the gorges must happen a normal of once every week more than a quarter of a year.

## What are causes, triggers, or hazard factors for emotional eating?

Like most emotional manifestations, emotional eating is believed to be the aftereffect of various factors as opposed to one single reason. A few explore is reliable with young ladies and ladies being at higher hazard for eating issue, demonstrating they are at higher hazard for emotional eating. Nonetheless, other research demonstrates that in certain populaces, men are bound to eat because of feeling discouragement or outrage, and ladies were bound to eat unnecessarily because of bombing an eating routine. It is believed that the expansion in the hormone cortisol that is one of the body's reactions to push is like the drug prednisone in its belongings. Specifically, both will in general trigger the body's pressure reaction, including expanded heart and breathing rate, blood flow to muscles, and visual keenness. Some portion of the pressure reaction regularly incorporates expanded hunger to supply the body with the fuel it needs to fight or flee, bringing about longings for supposed solace nourishments. Individuals who have been exposed to incessant as opposed to flitting pressure (like employment, school, or family stress, introduction to wrongdoing or misuse) are in danger of having constantly significant levels of cortisol in their bodies, adding to creating constant emotional-eating designs. Mentally, individuals who will in general interface nourishment with comfort, power, positive sentiments, or for some other reasons than giving fuel to their body can be inclined to emotional eating. They may eat to ¦ll an emotional void, when genuinely full, and take part in thoughtless eating. A few individuals whose feelings cause them to eat may have been raised to interface nourishment with sentiments rather than sustenance, especially if nourishment was rare or frequently utilized a prize or discipline, or as a substitute for emotional closeness.

**What are cautioning indications of emotional eating?**

Cautioning finishes paperwork for emotional eating incorporate a propensity to feel hunger strongly and out of nowhere, instead of bit by bit as happens with a genuine physical need to eat that is brought about by a vacant stomach. Emotional eaters will in general hunger for shoddy nourishments instead of trying to eat adjusted dinners, and the desire to eat is generally gone before by pressure or an awkward feeling or something to that affect, similar to fatigue, pity, outrage, blame, or dissatisfaction. Different signs of emotional eating are that the sufferer may feel an absence of control while eating and frequently feels remorseful for what they have eaten.

**What sort of masters treat emotional eating?**

Various distinctive social insurance experts assess and treat emotional eating and may likewise help with weight reduction when this adds to overweight or corpulence. As this side effect can happen at almost whenever over the life expectancy, everybody from pediatricians, family specialists, and other essential consideration doctors may address this issue. Medical attendants, nurture experts, and doctor associates might be associated with thinking about emotional-eating sufferers. Psychological well-being experts who are frequently associated with evaluating and treating this issue incorporate specialists, clinical analysts, social laborers, and authorized instructors. While any of these experts may think about individuals who take part in emotional eating, more than one may cooperate to enable the individual to beat this indication.

## How do medicinal services suppliers analyze emotional eating?

The finding of emotional eating is made after first guaranteeing that the sufferer has had a physical assessment and lab work to be sure that the side effect isn't a piece of some hereditary or other ailment like Prader-Willi disorder. As a feature of the emotional wellness part of the assessment, the patient might be posed a progression of inquiries from an institutionalized poll or individual test to help evaluate the nearness of emotional eating. Careful investigation of any history of psychological well-being side effects will be directed with the end goal that emotional eating can be recognized from other eating issue like bulimia, pigging out, or pica. An emotional wellness expert will likewise investigate whether other types of dysfunctional behavior are available.

## What is the treatment for emotional eating?

Defeating emotional eating will in general include showing the sufferer more advantageous approaches to see nourishment and grow better eating propensities, perceive their triggers for taking part right now, create fitting approaches to forestall and lighten pressure. A significant advance in overseeing pressure is work out, since normal physical action will in general hose the creation of stress synthetic compounds, even prompting a decline in wretchedness, uneasiness, and sleep deprivation notwithstanding diminishing the inclination to take part in emotional eating. Taking part in contemplation and other unwinding systems is additionally an incredible method to oversee pressure and in this manner decline emotional eating.

Along these lines, taking part in a couple of contemplation meetings daily can have enduring beneficialimpacts on wellbeing, in any event, diminishing high blood weight and pulse. Forgoing drug use and expending close to direct measures of liquor are other significant approaches to effectively oversee worry since a considerable lot of these substances increase the body's reaction to stretch. Additionally, enjoying utilization of those substances regularly forestalls the individual from confronting their issues straightforwardly so they are not ready to create compelling approaches to adapt to or dispense with the pressure.

Other way of life changes that can diminish pressure incorporate taking breaks at home and grinding away. Abstain from over-booking yourself. Figure out how to perceive and react to your pressure triggers. Take ordinary vacation days at interims that are directly for you. Structure your life to accomplish a agreeable approach to react to the unforeseen.

For the individuals who may require help managing pressure, stress-the executives guiding as individual or gathering treatment can be very valuable. Stress directing and bunch treatment have demonstrated to decrease pressure indications and improve generally wellbeing. Intellectual social treatment (CBT) has been seen as viable as a major aspect of treatment for fighting emotional eating. This methodology assists with lightening worry by helping the individual change their perspective about specific issues. In CBT, the advisor utilizes three procedures to achieve these objectives:

Educational segment: This stage assists with setting up inspirational desires for treatment and advance the individual's collaboration with the treatment procedure.

Psychological segment: This assists with distinguishing the contemplations and suppositions that influence the person's practices, especially those that may incline the sufferer to emotional eating. A variety of the psychological part of treatment is instructing care, giving nonjudgmental consideration to the present minute. Care includes thinking all the more reflectively, expanding one's emotional mindfulness, and will in general lead to an expanded capacity to isolate one's feelings from hunger.

Conduct part: This utilizes conduct modification strategies to show the individual how to stop emotional eating and utilize increasingly successful methodologies for managing issues.

On the off chance that pressure creates an out and out mental issue, as posttraumatic stress issue (PTSD), clinical wretchedness, or nervousness issue, at that point psychotropic meds, especially the particular serotonin reuptake inhibitors (SSRIs), can be amazingly valuable. Instances of SSRIs incorporate sertraline, (Zoloft), paroxetine (Paxil), §uoxetine (Prozac), citalopram (Celexa), or escitalopram (Lexapro).

Overeaters' Anonymous is a longstanding self improvement gathering that can be a significant asset for creating more beneficial approaches to see nourishment and perceiving and adapting to triggers for participating in emotional eating. Nutritionists, advisors, and other care groups can be other important assets.

**What is the visualization of emotional eating?**

Left untreated, emotional overeating can prompt confusions, as difficulties accomplishing weight reduction, stoutness, and even to the improvement of nourishment fixation. Then again, individuals who are inclined to emotional eating are likewise frequently increasingly receptive to stretch decrease in remedying their propensity to emotionally eat contrasted with people who will in general eat less when presented to pressure.

Is it conceivable to forestall emotional eating?

The anticipation of emotional eating basically includes decreasing pressure, utilizing productive approaches to comprehend and oversee feelings, and by utilizing nourishment as sustenance instead of an approach to take care of issues (eating to live as opposed to living to eat). Research additionally shows that reasoning about the future instead of remaining concentrated on fulfilling nourishment desires will in general forestall emotional eating. Different approaches to forestall emotional eating practices remember connecting with for contemplation, work out, and other useful pressure counteraction and stress the executives systems, as well as staying away from caffeine, liquor, or medications.

Halting Surface Behaviors: Why Diets Don't Work and Why It's Not About the Food Healing nourishment, weight, and self-perception issues, which are regularly deep rooted, isn't about simply eating better nourishment or being progressively dynamic, regardless of what the specialists state. It requires a methodology that makes you stride by-step through the pieces of yourself that are answerable for the start and continuation of your battles with weight, nourishment, and self-perception issues: your practices, your feelings, your convictions, and your relationship with your body and with nourishment. The objective of making these strides is for you to have the option to "clean house," to expel the things that never again fit your present life that may have been remaining from before. Right now, will address the practices that keep your weight what's more, nourishment issues set up and how to realign those practices with your real self and with how you need to live at this point.

Issues with nourishment or weight resemble an icy mass. Everybody can see the ice that is above the outside of the water, however they can't generally observe the bigger piece of the icy mass that is underneath the water. What stands out enough to be noticed is what's over the surface—weight, eating practices, for example, gorging or overeating, and body disappointment. These practices can make your life unmanageable, creating money related hardships, clinical issues, and general despondency. Your nourishment and self-perception issues and the related practices are what stands out enough to be noticed in light of the fact that they are what you are centered around, what your companions what's more, family realize that you stress over, and what assume control over your life. Envision what your life would resemble on the off chance that you didn't invest a large portion of your energy contemplating your weight, how to get more fit, what you resemble, how embarrassed you are of your body, what you're arranging to eat or what you are attempting to shield yourself from eating, etc.

You might be understanding this and thinking, My weight is the most significant issue. On the off chance that I could simply get thinner, I wouldn't have an issue. In the event that you put your emphasis on the number on the scale and all the practices you use to attempt to change that number, you will pass up on the chance for mending at the most profound level conceivable. Genuine recuperating requires not just that you get to what is superficially however that you search for and recuperate the main driver of your nourishment and weight issues, which as a rule lies underneath the surface (and isn't as self-evident). Weight and nourishment issues are simply indications of the more concerning issue. Consequently, just tending to the weight or eating issue doesn't influence the more profound issues of feelings that might be wild and cause you to gorge, of convictions that are oblivious however are driving the eating practices, what's more, of an absence of association with your body's intrinsic intelligence, which can assist you with your eating and weight issues. An individual can quit gorging or cleansing yet at the same time be helpless before more profound convictions, feelings, and distractions that remove him from all he really needs access his life, including joy and significant serenity. Underneath the surface are solid and at times difficult feelings, center convictions, and body impressions that drive these practices. These Halting Surface Behaviors shallow practices are an approach to keep these amazing and now and again terrifying feelings what's more, convictions under control. For instance, Billy utilized nourishment as an approach to adapt to pity and despondency. Just as for Billy's situation, just tending to the shallow layer with abstaining from excessive food intake or even bariatric medical procedure won't take care of the basic issues and will prompt the weight being recaptured.

**Shallow Behaviors**

The eating practices at the shallow level incorporate overeating; gorging; abstaining from excessive food intake; the utilization of diet pills, diuretics, or intestinal medicines; cleansing; and emotional overeating. Different practices that can be placed right now illicit drug use, liquor abuse, sex habit, and love and relationship enslavement. While these last practices may not be explicitly nourishment related, they regularly co-happen with weight and self-perception issues.

The initial step to recuperating is figuring out how to stop the practices, which will give you the space to recoup what your identity is (your true self) and to figure out how to comprehend and adapt to upsetting feelings in manners that don't include nourishment.

**Changing Superficial Behaviors**

Similarly as icy masses come in numerous shapes and sizes, you may discover your response to tending to your weight, self-perception, and nourishment issues will appear in a wide range of structures.

Now and then what's superficially appears to be so enormous and overpowering ("How am I going to lose one hundred pounds?!") that you may feel like you are remaining on the edge of a precipice and are startled of bouncing off. In different cases, what's superficially may appear to be something that isn't too difficult to even think about doing ("I've shed pounds previously; I can do it once more"), however when you start to look further—

at what's underneath the surface, at the feelings driving your practices, at past damages and injuries, or even at center convictions you've held dear the vast majority of your life—you become dreadful and overpowered and can't oversee a way. The two responses are typical and not unforeseen.

You may likewise find that you have a double or clashed relationship with these practices. For instance, you may perceive that specific nourishments don't cause you to feel great however that you can't quit eating them. You may gorge on sugary nourishments toward the evening, at that point feel wiped out and tired the majority of the remainder of the day just to wind up needing to gorge again later in the evening. Eating certain nourishments might be soothing yet may bring about sentiments of blame and disgrace a short time later. This is the double relationship. As you work through this book, you will find different approaches to solace or support yourself. As a feature of setting yourself up to stop these practices, it will assist you with becoming increasingly mindful of how nourishment came to speak to adore, solace, security, or whatever it as of now speaks to you. Until you can distinguish the unique association that you manufactured with nourishment, you will experience issues breaking the cycle that keeps you stuck on the grounds that your psyche may think you need to eat on the grounds that you are eager while your feelings are driving you to eat on account of tragically deceased recollections associating explicit nourishments to love, solace, or security. This mindfulness will clarify why you couldn't stop gorging on specific nourishments or why you end up overeating to the point of feeling debilitated despite the fact that you would prefer truly not to. As we experience the initial five sections, you will begin making these associations.

Alert: If you wind up feeling overpowered or stuck whenever during this procedure, you may need to go after help. Backing can come as expert assistance from an advisor, or you may feel bolstered by connecting with a companion or relative.

Exercise: Identifying Your Behaviors Checkmark all the practices that may have some relationship to your weight or to how you feel about nourishment and your body.

> bingeing (eating a huge amount of nourishment in a brief timeframe, typically two hours or less)
> hiding or accumulating nourishment
> eating covertly
> emotional eating
> overeating under pressure
> overeating when tired
> using diet pills, purgatives, or water pills (diuretics)
> not eating throughout the day (limiting)
> stealing nourishment
> using illicit medications to deal with your hunger
> dieting

## Do I Really Need to Eat That?

All that you do, including your eating practices and why you eat what you eat, and how you feel about your body, occurs which is as it should be. It's known as the shallow level in light of the fact that while it is an issue, it isn't the underlying driver—it's exactly what is nearest to the surface. Nourishment isn't the issue. It's the manner by which you use nourishment that causes issues. In the event that you just location practices, change will be brief. It is important to burrow further—to look underneath the surface—to comprehend what drives you to utilize nourishment the manner in which you do.

Frequently the practices that are a piece of the shallow level began when you were more youthful be that as it may, just got troublesome as you got more established. These practices may have been gone before by occasions throughout your life that you presumably have not contemplated in years and may not interface to your present issues with weight.

Beneficial encounters assume a key job in the advancement and propagation of eating and weight issues. Troublesome beneficial encounters can frequently create turmoil between eating for sustenance and eating only for delight. This can lead us to persuade ourselves that we need to treat, prize, or solace ourselves with nourishment.

Eating conduct is constrained by the mind, which directions appetite and totality prompts with data sent from the stomach related tract. One piece of the cerebrum (the nerve center) controls the need to eat for endurance that is inalienable in every living being. An alternate part of the cerebrum controls our longing to eat. This piece of the mind is known as the dopamine reward focus. Regularly the need to eat for endurance can be superseded by our longing for a specific taste or then again a specific nourishment. This is the thing that can prompt stoutness. In days of yore, when nourishment was more diligently to acquire and there were no drive-through joints, there was no weight. On the off chance that you lived during those occasions, you had quite recently enough nourishment to address your body's issues however once in a while more than that.

In present day times, there is a bounty of nourishment, and nourishment is substantially more effectively accessible. There are cafés, inexpensive food places, supermarkets, etc. So except if you live in a creating nation or you are amazingly poor, you will have enough nourishment to eat. Eating past your requirement for nourishment for the most part implies eating solace food sources that are regularly high in sugar, fat, and salt. These nourishments are eaten not for their dietary benefit however for their taste, to fulfill emotional longings, or to adapt to pressure. There is nothing amiss with eating delectable treats, yet your failure to forego these nourishments or to stop enthusiastically overeating them is a sign you might be utilizing such nourishments for their taste as well as for emotional reasons. Individuals devour these nourishments in any event, when they are not eager and regularly without pondering what they are eating and here and there without getting a charge out of what they are eating. It is essential to intrude on this cycle so as to deal with your weight.

## Why Diets Don't Work

On the off chance that you are overweight, you might be inspired to count calories and get in shape for some significant reasons—for better wellbeing and prosperity, for expanded versatility, to be all the more socially acknowledged, and to abstain from being prodded or harassed about your weight. You may likewise accept that getting in shape will take care of different issues throughout your life, for example, feeling disengaged, needing a relationship, or needing to excel busy working. Getting more fit can deliver a brief inclination of satisfaction just to be supplanted without anyone else fault, gloom, or sadness when you are not capable to keep up your weight reduction. It has become some portion of our way of life to utilize diets to get in shape what's more, when they don't work, to reprimand ourselves for "not staying with it."

In spite of the way that reviews show consumes less calories don't bring about manageable weight reduction, you may resemble most of overweight people who despite everything accept that abstaining from excessive food intake is a successful weight reduction system (Thomas et al. 2008). Not exclusively accomplish slims down not work, yet in the event that you've been eating fewer carbs now and again for an amazing duration, you may have seen, as one investigation appears, that you've recaptured more weight than you've lost, which is the experience of 66% of weight watchers in considers (Mann et al. 2007). One of the issues that numerous substantial people face is that they've been told again and again that on the off chance that they don't get thinner, they can't be solid. While this might be an impermanent inspiration that has helped you diet previously, having the attention on your weight doesn't really change your wellbeing. You are more liable to improve your wellbeing in the event that you center around changing your practices, instead of on the number on the scale. Studies bolster that when you put your emphasis on wellbeing first, not weight, you're bound to improve your wellbeing, confidence, and self-perception and lower your hazard for coronary illness, hypertension, and diabetes through size acknowledgment, natural eating, and expanded action levels (Bacon and Aphramor 2011).

On the off chance that plainly eats less carbs don't work, for what reason do a great many people hold going to the most recent trend diet, trusting that each time things will be unique? The appropriate response is that each diet speaks to a trust they have of transforming them. In our fat-phobic, diet-fixated culture, we have come to mistake being meager for being glad. We have been adapted to accept that we need to look a specific route so as to merit the existence we need. We have been instructed by the media, our families, and society that on the off chance that we are in a greater body—or in the event that we are diverse in any capacity from what society considers adequate (youthful, slender, not gay, of a specific race or then again religion or political connection)— that we can't have what others have and, most significantly, what we urgently need.

Every one of us has inside us a yearning for our best life, for our fantasy life. Is befuddling that we have likened shallow characteristics of appearance and size, for instance, with what they speak to for us in our best life. For instance, on the off chance that you trust you must be slight so as to have the relationship you long for, you may have overlooked what you're truly yearning for, which is the inclination of personal association and how that would fill your heart.

In the event that you have not had the option to arrive at your weight objective, you may have shut yourself to any possibility of that event except if and until you are flimsy. Fundamentally, dreams are deferred or on the other hand even shut down, hanging tight for you to have your ideal body. In the following activity, you'll list the fantasies you've been requiring to be postponed until you are slender.

Right now, will find out about the shrouded power that is driving your practices and what you can do to uncouple your practices from the feelings that drive them. These emotional drivers originate from past encounters and convictions, from old injuries that have never mended, and from current encounters that recreate old emotional examples. You will additionally figure out how to recognize emotional reactions that are not consistent with whom you are today. Some portion of changing your practices is understanding the more profound main thrusts behind them. When you become mindful of how feelings can trigger some practices, you will have a superior possibility of reacting to your feelings in a manner that doesn't include utilizing nourishment to numb yourself from the torment of your feelings, push them down, or overlook them. Right now, will likewise find out about emotional examples that may have begun in youth and how those might be influencing your current-day responses. Maryann's story above, for instance, shows how individuals throughout her life, beginning with her mom and now her better half, have concentrated on her weight. The feelings she feels about this began in her adolescence, and now, as a grown-up, these equivalent feelings are activated when her significant other offers remarks about her weight or absence of wellness. The feelings of humiliation, blame, disgrace, outrage, depression, and frustration are the driving power behind her overeating.

On the off chance that you resemble numerous individuals with nourishment and weight issues, you might have the option to perceive that your feelings now and again feel overpowering, or you might be the kind of individual who has totally shut down any entrance to your feelings and even experiences difficulty recognizing what you are feeling. The two responses to emotional torment are cut out of the same cloth—endeavorsto escape from your feelings, or from the "emotional soup." When you are stuck in the emotional soup, you may feel that your feelings are responsible for you instead of the other path around. Rising up out of the emotional soup requires emotional improvement— that is, having the option to distinguish, express, comprehend, and critically, control your feelings. It isn't your feelings themselves that mess up your life. Or maybe it is your endeavor to smother or evade your feelings that prompts issues. At the point when feelings are not recognized, they discover articulation in the nourishments you eat, in the size and state of your body, and in the need to eat nourishments that might be mitigating immediately however don't extinguish the spirit's strive after articulation. Emotional guideline implies having the option to adapt with feelings without depending on undesirable or reckless practices. Numerous elements that impact emotional advancement and particularly emotional guideline will be examined right now. Above all, I'd prefer to discuss what feelings are and why they are so significant in our lives.

**What Are Emotions?**

Feelings can be characterized as "inner marvels that can, yet don't generally, make themselves discernible through articulation and conduct" (Niedenthal, Krauth-Gruber, and Ric 2006, 5). Webster's word reference characterizes a feeling as "a cognizant mental response (as outrage or dread) emotionally experienced as solid inclination normally coordinated toward a particular object and commonly joined by physiological and conduct changes in the body" (Merriam-Webster Online, s.v. "feeling"). The Taoist perspective on feelings is that they are vitality. Feelings can be known as the vitality of self-articulation. How we communicate emotionally turns out to be a piece of how others distinguish us and frequently how we consider ourselves. Feelings can likewise impact our discernments. For instance, in the event that you hear a canine yelping, contingent upon your past experience and impression of canines, you may attempt to pet the pooch. On the off chance that then again, your past encounters with hounds have been negative and prompted a dread of hounds or if the pooch appears to be undermining, you might need to abstain from drawing near to the canine. Feelings can be the sign that can draw us toward what we like and caution us away from threat. On account of a canine woofing, observation halfway decides how you see the circumstance. Be that as it may, the feeling of dread at the sound of a pooch woofing can likewise be an indication of genuine risk. The precarious part is sifting through what is recognition and what is genuine peril. Frequently past encounters make it hard for us to perceive what is genuine, and right now will study the effect of understanding on observation and how it can shading reality.

Feelings can likewise assist you with settling on choices throughout your life. Individuals who have had harm to the emotional pieces of the mind think that its troublesome, if certainly feasible, to decide. On the off chance that you have had harm to your emotional mind, you may experience difficulty making even straightforward choices, for example, what to eat (Bechara, Damasio, and Damasio 2000). People and most different creatures are outfitted with a fundamental arrangement of center feelings: dread, outrage, shock, appall, euphoria, and misery (Ekman, Friesen, and Ellsworth 1982). People additionally have a lot of higher good feelings that are subject to our degree of reluctance also, capacity to relate to other people. These incorporate blame, humiliation, disgrace, and pride (Leary and Price 2012).

Later right now, will talk about emotional guideline finally. Be that as it may, next, I'd prefer to focus on different parts of emotional improvement—the capacity to recognize, acknowledge, what's more, express your feelings.

**Distinguishing Emotions**

There are numerous manners by which we can perceive feelings in ourselves and in others. Infants impart their feelings nonverbally from birth through crying, facial articulations, and body stances. At the point when a parent peruses these nonverbal prompts and reacts properly, it makes a sentiment of security and wellbeing for the newborn child. Figuring out how to recognize feelings in others happens when we are youthful. How every one of us figures out how to recognize feelings changes incredibly. As a kid, you may have been instructed about feelings through discussions about upsetting circumstances. For instance, on the off chance that you got back home from school and your mom saw you were disturbed, she may have requested that you distinguish your feelings: "Jimmy, are you irate about something that occurred at school?" However, you may have experienced childhood in a home where when you got back home from school upset, no one paid consideration or you were told, "Quit moping and go to your room." If along these lines, you may have learned that your feelings don't make a difference. On the off chance that you were abused or mishandled as a kid, you may have figured out how to fear your feelings since demonstrating feelings could prompt further misuse. Also, feelings may have been terrifying to you as a kid in the event that you have a hereditary inclination to having exceptionally serious emotional reactions or to being touchy to your own or others' feelings.

In the event that you are not ready to recognize your feelings or the feelings of others, you may discover yourself in circumstances that are perilous. For instance, if a chime goes off in school, the instructor shows that she is apprehensive, and different children start to feel dread as well, yet you don't pick up on the prompt, you may not understand that you have to leave the structure rapidly as a result of a fire. Another motivation behind why it's essential to distinguish your feelings is that else you won't have an approach to name your inner experience. You may feel horrendous however not know why what's more, not have the option to plainly communicate what "terrible" signifies to you. Does feeling terrible mean you're apprehensive or tired? Or on the other hand does it mean you're discouraged? Having the option to recognize your feelings is a piece of what permits you to communicate as a person. At long last, on the off chance that you have been hereditarily inclined to having extremely serious feelings yet can't distinguish what you are feeling, you may feel overpowered by them and simply shut down or numb yourself—with nourishment, for instance.

Outward appearances are a significant nonverbal approach to distinguish feelings. The articulations used to pass on seven general feelings—outrage, trouble, shock, scorn, disturb, dread, and euphoria—are comparative all through the world (Matsumoto et al. 2008). In Western culture, researchers have had the option to delineate one feelings that individuals use nearly precisely the same outward appearances for, including blend feelings, for example, "joyfully astounded" (Du, Tao, and Martinez 2014). Other nonverbal emotional prompts can incorporate body stance and hand motions. On the off chance that you are corpulent, you may likewise experience experienced issues perceiving nonverbal prompts of feelings from others or come up short on the capacity to portray and recognize your own feelings, a condition called alexithymia, which will in general be higher in fat kids and grown-ups and ladies with binge-eating issue (Baldaro et al. 2003; Pinaquy et al. 2003). This means fat ladies who experience issues imparting their sentiments additionally are bound to eat in light of their feelings. The specific reasons for alexithymia are not known, however it might be the aftereffect of youth misuse or may occur as a protection component, a method for adapting to past encounters of extreme what's more, overpowering emotional encounters (McDougall 1989).

Powerlessness to recognize feelings in oneself or others may likewise be a reason for emotional overeating, particularly in men (Larsen et al. 2006). On the off chance that you are a lady, you are most likely more exact than most men at distinguishing feelings from nonverbal signals, for example, facial articulations. It might be that ladies are associated at a prior age to distinguish nonverbal emotional prompts, or it might be that the female mind is simply modified for this ability (Hall also, Matsumoto 2004). There is a scope of approaches to communicate emotionally. Some are more advantageous than others. However, before you can communicate your feelings, you should turn out to be more mindful of them. You should have the option to recognize what feeling you are feeling. In the activity underneath, invest some energy figuring out how to recognize your feelings.

**Emotional Expression**

Figuring out how to recognize your feelings, to put a name to what you are feeling, is the first venture to having the option to communicate feelings in a sound and safe manner. Emotional articulation is significant in light of the fact that it permits you to be the individual you are, with your own discernments, feelings, and perspectives. Emotional articulation additionally is a vital piece of what it implies to be human.

Regardless of whether you didn't experience childhood in a broken home, the messages you found out about step by step instructions to deal with your feelings—for instance which feelings were viewed as fitting in which circumstances—may have originated from your family's social foundation. There may have additionally been social guidelines about the sorts of occasions in which emotional articulation was authorized. In numerous societies, for instance, crying as a declaration of pain over the demise of a friend or family member is viewed as typical.

Examples of emotional articulation may likewise be like examples in your relationship with nourishment. For instance, you may skip dinners (like retention feelings), which normally sets you up for the following binge (or emotional upheaval).

Numerous individuals experience difficulty communicating certain feelings—typically in light of the fact that they have a judgment about themselves (or feel others will pass judgment on them) on the off chance that they feel certain emotions. For model, you may feel that you will be decided as being feeble on the off chance that you express trouble. Emotional articulation must go connected at the hip with emotional guideline, which you will find out about later right now. Until further notice, in the activity beneath, check whether you can discover any connections to your eating practices and your feelings.

**How Could You Learn to Express Your Emotions?**

Every family has designs, frequently implicit, concerning feelings. You may not recollect explicit principles being discussed, yet the standards were the manner in which you figured out how to communicate your feelings— either legitimately or in a roundabout way. Emotional guidelines can incorporate ones that (1) permit a kid to change their demeanor of specific feelings to secure someone else's sentiments and (2) cover feelings to shield oneself from hurt or to maintain a strategic distance from shame (Saarni 1999). For instance, your mom might not have let you know not to get irate, however she may have left the room or given you an objecting look at whatever point you communicated outrage, showing that communicating outrage was inadmissible. Or on the other hand your dad may have hollered at you, "Don't you sass me," when you blew up, recommending that it was not alright for you to blow up or express that outrage, yet that it was alright for him to do as such.

Notice that feelings themselves are not terrible or wrong. In some casesmessages you get the hang of growing up may lead you to either adhere to family administers about feelings or on the other hand betray them reflexively. You may likewise have decisions about past encounters and the feelings related with those encounters. These decisions and related feelings are what keep you stuck in a story (experience) from quite a while ago. Re-encountering the feelings that are kept set up by your judgment of past encounters is a reason for overeating what's more, gorging. For instance, on the off chance that you resented your ex during your separation procedures, you may have a judgment that he is a terrible individual or a "yank" since he hurt you. Each time you see him, that judgment may come up for you—"he's a twitch"—and you may feel furious and hurt once more. On the off chance that you clutch this judgment and keep on remaining irate about what occurred during that time, you are stuck in a past that never again exists right now. You may feel extremely supported about your indignation in light of the fact that your exhusband accomplished something that hurt you. In any case, ask yourself whom your judgment and your outrage toward him are truly stinging. Is it accurate to say that they are harming him? Presumably not. They are harming you. They are causing languishing over you. At the point when you keep on returning and live in a past experience as though it's happening in your present, it will affect numerous regions of your life and your connections—with your ex as well as likely with others in your life who may help you to remember him or help you to remember how he affected you. Holding on to decisions about past encounters can likewise influence your longing to indulge as an approach to numb an inclination that is actually a relic from quite a while ago. All things being equal, you are not the same individual who experienced that experience, and clutching it just adds to enduring (and presumably overeating or gorging) presently. To discharge yourself from the annoyance and damages of the past, you need to quit making a decision about your ex. This isn't to imply that you overlook your hurt emotions; rather, you advise yourself that the hurt is from the past, and you find ways, maybe in therapy, to work through past damages so you can live more completely in the present. At the point when you clutch the judgment, "He's an awful individual since he hurt me," for model, you keep yourself detained by the feelings related with that old circumstance, instead of being the onlooker and on-screen character in your present life. Doing this isn't simple, yet at the point when you can see that clutching the past just damages you, you may find that it turns out to be progressively significant for you to travel through the past and embrace current circumstances. By discharging yourself from these decisions, you may get yourself progressively open to the full range of emotional articulation accessible to us as individuals.

**Emotional Regulation**

So as to utilize feelings, it is essential to realize how to oversee or manage them without utilizing nourishment. Maryann's story above is a genuine case of an emotional overeater—somebody who utilizes nourishment to manage her feelings. Emotional guideline starts in early outset when infants figure out how to self-mitigate or quiet themselves. Around 20 percent of infants give indications of trouble with self-guideline through over the top crying, rest, and taking care of issues or attentional issue (Schmid et al. 2010). For most, this is a transitory issue. Be that as it may, for a few, this might be an indication of what might be on the horizon. By the age of four, kids have typically figured out how to change how they express feelings to suit the desires for other people—they've taken in the social and family leads about emotional articulation as examined previously. Most youngsters keep on learning different self-guideline abilities as they get more seasoned. They may learn, for instance, to communicate negative feelings more frequently to their mom than their dad, who may respond all the more contrarily to emotional presentations. They may figure out how to occupy themselves by running on the play area when they feel on edge.

You might be utilizing numerous solid methods for directing your feelings in different territories of your life at the same time, as Maryann, end up at a misfortune going to how to do that with weight, body disappointment, and nourishment issues. For instance, Maryann needs to direct her feelings in her fill in as a medical caretaker, where it may not be fitting for her to communicate how she feels to her patients, however she can communicate those sentiments to a colleague. While everybody gorges from time to time (Thanksgiving, for instance), when you use nourishment as your essential method for managing your feelings, it can not just compound negative feelings, for example, blame what's more, disgrace, yet in addition lead to weight gain and ensuing body disappointment. Some portion of what you will learn right now how to manage your feelings so you don't need to utilize nourishment as an unfortunate method for managing them. The objective is to have the option to encounter an ordinary scope of feelings without feeling so awkward with those feelings that you use nourishment (or on the other hand different substances or practices) to abstain from managing them.

**Why Is Emotional Regulation Important?**
Emotional overeating practices are the aftereffect of poor emotional guideline systems what's more, aptitudes, including the capacity to distinguish and adapt to feelings (Haedt-Matt and Keel 2011; Ricca et al. 2009). On the off chance that you are an emotional overeater, this issue presumably started from the get-go in your life. As a kid, on the off chance that you experienced difficulty dealing with your feelings, this was a sign that you were at higher

hazard for being overweight or large as a grown-up. Or on the other hand in the event that you experienced issues deferring satisfaction as a youngster, pitched fits, or communicated exorbitant resentment about nourishment, this likewise would have put you in danger for weight and nourishment issues (Agras et al. 2004; Seeyave et al. 2009).

Curiously, on the off chance that you are an individual who experiences issues simply tolerating your sentiments and being emotionally disturbed makes it difficult for you to think, center, total undertakings, or work obligations, you may likewise be bound to battle with nourishment and weight issues (Gianini, White, and Masheb 2013; Sim and Zeman 2006). At the point when your feelings are in control, the outcomes can be grave—for your connections and absolutely for your relationship with nourishment and your body.

While eating in light of emotional triggers or negative states of mind is regular in numerous with weight issues, you may have seen that the negative feelings don't leave after you binge or indulge. Overeating may unknowingly be your method for attempting to change those negative emotions. Be that as it may, ask yourself to what extent you get alleviation after a binge or after emotionally overeating. You may begin eating in light of outrage just to discover your annoyance still there after your binge. Just presently, you're irate with yourself for eating that pack of chips! In addition, you may then feel humiliated and remorseful about the binge. The point is utilizing nourishment to oversee feelings is simply not the best methodology. It might have been something you realized when you were a youngster and didn't generally have different aptitudes, yet presently you do, and you will figure out how to take advantage of other ranges of abilities for emotional guideline.

## WHY CANT I MANAGE MY EMOTIONS?

Numerous people with weight issues or eating issue learn at a youthful age to stifle all or certain feelings. You may have been shown this straightforwardly, or you may have taken in this message in a roundabout way through experience or perception. On the off chance that each time you got irritated as a kid you were told, "Be a decent young lady," or "Young men don't cry," after some time you may have underestimated this is the manner by which you ought to carry on. Or on the other hand you may have had a parent who was a seething heavy drinker and scared you. This could lead you to abstain from communicating your outrage since you might fear turning out to resemble your alcoholic parent. This adolescence experience can appear in adulthood as a dread of any individual who communicates outrage, regardless of whether it's a solid articulation of outrage by your life partner. This thusly could prompt staying away from any contention in your relationship, which isn't solid for you. Another situation right now the kid who relates to and copies the alcoholic parent, considering him to be her as the more grounded parent. This could prompt an acknowledgment of seething as the best approach to show quality in connections. In adulthood, she may turn into the individual who seethes, similarly as her dad or mother did when she was growing up.

Another explanation you may experience issues with your feelings may have to do with explicit sorts of encounters from your adolescence, as indicated by the Adverse Childhood Encounters (ACE) Study. In the event that you encountered verbal, physical, or sexual maltreatment, if a part of your family was in prison, on the off chance that one of your folks was intellectually sick or mishandling medications or liquor, or on the other hand if your folks were separated or your mom was a casualty of abusivebehavior at home, your hazard of having a weight issue (characterized as having a weight file [BMI] more prominent than or equivalent to 35kg/m2) might be 46 percent higher than it is for individuals who didn't have these impeding youth encounters (Brown et al. 2009; Felitti et al. 1998). One of the specialists right now that "a large number of his patients had been unwittingly utilizing heftiness as a shield against undesirable sexual consideration or as a type of protection against physical assault, and that a significant number of them had been explicitly or potentially truly mishandled as kids.

In other words, despite the fact that stoutness was expectedly seen as the issue, it was regularly seen as the oblivious answer for other, unmistakably increasingly disguised, issues" (see http:// www.acestudy.org for more data; Anda and Felitti 2003, 1). Misuse or disregard or any of the above negative encounters in youth prompts what is called dangerous pressure. Harmful pressure prompts an overproduction of the pressure hormones, cortisol, adrenaline, and noradrenaline. This prompts physical harm to the cerebrum. In the event that you were a youngster who experienced harmful pressure, at that point you carried on with your life in battle flight-or-freeze mode.

Everything on the planet may have appeared to be risky or perilous to you. This could have made you battle or fall behind in a difficult situation creating solid associations with companions and educators because of your failure to confide in others, or you may have encountered a feeling of basic despondency and dissatisfaction for a mind-blowing duration. Individuals who have had harmful worry in their life frequently discover comfort in nourishment, medications, or liquor; wrong sex; high-hazard sports; or work as an approach to adapt to their sentiments of sorrow, dread, and disgrace. That is the reason overeating and stoutness are not about nourishment or about weight. Or maybe, the weight and overeating are an answer that you utilized when you were more youthful and didn't have the abilities you have now, however they are not the issue. The issue has to do with poisonous stress and what caused it.

## Connection Style and Expressing Emotions

Research is presently indicating that something many refer to as "connection styles" may likewise clarify why individuals with a background marked by lethal pressure identified with youth injury or to other explicit youth issues (surrender, disregard, unexpected division from a parent, visit changes in guardians, or absence of parental figure responsiveness) may have weight and nourishment issues. Your parent or essential guardian's responsiveness or affectability to your requirements from early stages decides your own connection style. Infants append to individuals who are touchy and responsive in social associations with them and who are reliably in their lives between ages a half year and two years. As a newborn child figures out how to creep and afterward walk, he utilizes his guardians and other recognizable individuals throughout his life as a safe base from which to investigate his condition, knowing whether he runs into any issues, he can come back to that protected base for solace and wellbeing (Waters and Cummings 2000). You will get familiar with connection styles in the following section. Until further notice, you would realize that you had a safe connection style as a kid (and maybe now) in the event that you had a sense of security to draw in with outsiders, were vexed when your mother left you, and were glad when she returned. You would likewise have felt as though your world was a protected spot for you to investigate and realize that on the off chance that you required assistance, you could turn to your mom or essential guardian.

Secure newborn children figure out how to confide in their emotions, and they additionally figure out how to confide in their perspective on the world, which begins from their folks or guardians. Some portion of the emotional advancement of secure newborn children is figuring out how to portray and convey their feelings. Secure youngsters invest more energy communicating physical and emotional requirements than do kids who have been abused. On the off chance that you encountered any of the youth encounters referenced in the above area, you may think that its hard to control your emotions. You may have additionally experienced feelings uniquely in contrast to the remainder of your family, and this could likewise influence your connection style (De Schipper, Oosterman, and Schuengel2012). For instance, in some cases guardians who are exceptionally cordial may energize a bashful youngster to be more socially intuitive than she feels great with, where a progressively delicate parent would be all the more consoling and steady. Indeed, even without messages from the family, youngsters who are increasingly hindered may create approaches to oversee dread or nervousness that can later lead to overeating. After some time, for instance, a modest kid may keep on expelling herself from social circumstances and go to gorging or overeating, prompting weight issues, sorrow, and uneasiness (which worsen overeating) in later years. A family situation where there is a jumble between the earth and the kid's disposition, where a youngster's feelings are not approved by her folks or parental figures, or where emotional articulations are either overlooked or discredited can set the kid up for later weight and eating issues.

In the event that you experienced childhood in such a family, you figured out how to imagine that your view and experience of feelings is inaccurate (Linehan 1993). This at that point may have made you have issues with emotional guideline since you never figured out how to distinguish, express, what's more, control your feelings suitably. This is exceptionally relevant to your later issues with nourishment and eating as most people with eating issue (counting binge-eating clutter) say that they experience issues enduring forceful feelings and use nourishment to stay away from feeling or activating such compelling feelings or will utilize rash practices to oversee them (Corstorphine et al. 2007; Van der Kolk and Fisler 1994).

On the off chance that you experienced childhood in a home where you discovered that it isn't worthy or safe to communicate feelings, particularly negative ones, this could affect your eating practices in a few different ways: (1) you may have figured out how to "hinder" your familiarity with these "inadmissible" or then again refuted feelings through binge eating, cleansing (self-initiated retching), or selfharming practices, or (2) you may have figured out how to square feelings through habitual overeating, enthusiastic exercise, or confining your nourishment consumption (Mountford et al. 2007; Waller, Kennerley, and Ohanian 2007). People who were brought up in a family where their folks discredited their perspectives or emotions are bound to binge and cleanse or have other disarranged eating practices. On the off chance that your family put a ton of accentuation on accomplishment and achievement and the need to control one's feelings, you may have utilized urgent exercise as a method for managing your feelings (Haslam et al. 2008). Experiencing childhood in a negating condition could likewise be viewed as another youth experience that causes harmful stress.

In the activities beneath, check whether you identify with any of the encounters either in adolescence or adulthood, which can prompt issues with connection (unreliable connection). In the next part, you will study how these encounters can prompt explicit connection styles and how they can influence your weight and self-perception.

## COMPULSIVE EATING

### What is compulsive eating?

compulsive eating, likewise called binge eating, is portrayed by a solid, wild motivation to devour a lot of nourishment. At times, enthusiastic eating advances into binge eating issue (BED), which is a formal determination. In others, it happens just at explicit occasions, for example, during the days paving the way to your period.

- ✓ Some basic side effects of impulsive eating include:
- ✓ eating when you aren't ravenous or in any event, when you feel full
- ✓ frequently eating a lot of nourishment
- ✓ feeling resentful or embarrassed after a binge
- ✓ eating stealthily or eating continually for the duration of the day

Habitual eating portrays a conduct that is available with certain structures of eating issue. It's anything but a finding in its own right, yet to a greater degree a depiction of a kind of conduct. It is normally used to depict visit scenes of wild eating, where an individual keeps on eating nourishment long after they feel full and in some cases to the point of feeling debilitated. Individuals who take part in impulsive eating may meet criteria for Binge Eating Disorder. On the off chance that somebody cleanses after a binge by regurgitating, working out, utilizing intestinal medicines, diuretics, or purifications, they may meet criteria for Bulimia Nervosa. Both of these are eating clutter judgments and looking for treatment as quickly as time permits is significant.

The American Psychiatric Association distributes a manual for diagnosing emotional wellness issue. As indicated by that manual, called the DSM-5, for somebody to be determined to have Binge Eating Disorder they should meet the accompanying criteria:

Intermittent and tireless scenes of binge eating.

A binge scene happens during a timeframe (ex. 2 hours) during which the individual expends anmeasure of nourishment bigger than the vast majority would eat under comparable conditions. Experience lost power over eating during the binge scene.

A binge incorporates in any event three of the accompanying:

1) Eating quicker than expected
2) Eating past the purpose of agreeable totality
3) Eating a huge amount of nourishment in spite of not feeling hungry
4) Eating without anyone else to shroud the sum you're eating to keep away from judgment or feeling humiliated
5) Feeling disgrace, bitterness, blame, or nervousness after binge eating

Binge eating occurs at any rate once every week for 3 months or more. The binge isn't made up for, i.e there is no cleansing, overexercising, douche or purgative use. There is noteworthy trouble because of binge eating. Inflexible eating practices, for example, slimming down, discontinuous fasting, or removing nutrition classes have been connected to a higher occurrence of BED. Individuals who battle with negative self-perception may at first confine nourishment or diet in request to get more fit. This limitation in calories may then start a pattern of binge eating conduct as their body spirals out of equalization and endeavors to shield itself from "starvation". This confine binge cycle, alongside conceivable weight change, can be trailed by sentiments of weakness, blame, disgrace and disappointment. Going to nourishment can become a characteristic method to adapt to these troublesome emotions. Individuals who take part in enthusiastic eating ordinarily feel wild and know that their eating designs are anomalous Many accuse themselves and think in the event that they could simply control their nourishment allow or get thinner they. This site utilizes treats to improve your experience. We'll accept that you're satisfied with this, yet you can quit on the off chance that you wish irregular. Many accuse themselves and think in the event that they could simply control their nourishment allow or get more fit, they would feel good. This may make them become significantly increasingly prohibitive with nourishment. Shockingly, the more we attempt to control nourishment, the more nourishment begins to control us and it gets hard to end the limit binge shame cycle.

Binge Eating Disorder is the most widely recognized eating issue and is seen as a genuine emotional well-being condition. Like anorexia and bulimia, habitual eating can bring about mental what's more, clinical difficulties. Luckily, with appropriate assistance, this can be dealt with and individuals can heal.

It's prescribed to work with a treatment group that spends significant time in eating issue including an authorized advisor, enrolled dietitian, clinical specialist, and here and there a specialist. Inpatient and Intensive Outpatient treatment might be important to offer the best possible help. Get familiar with treatment.

Extra Signs and Symptoms to Look For Dread of not having the option to quit eating deliberately Sorrow, tension, irritability Self-expostulating contemplations following gorges Pulling back from exercises as a result of shame about weight or eating practices Going on a wide range of diets Distraction with nourishment Eating little in broad daylight or around others Accepting they will be a superior individual if their body changes Sentiments about self depend on weight Social and expert disappointments ascribed to weight Feeling tormented by eating propensities Weight is the focal point of life Emotional Eating

Emotional Eating is another term that is every now and again utilized yet isn't an eating issue determination. It alludes to examples when an individual goes to nourishment for comfort as opposed to hunger. By and large of emotional eating, the individual is under some type of pressure. Emotional eating can likewise allude to times when an individual uses nourishment as a reward, following a monotonous day grinding away, or when they feel forlorn or discouraged. Emotional yearning is not quite the same as physical appetite. It frequently goes ahead out of nowhere and feels like an earnest requirement for nourishment. Physical yearning tends to develop all the more step by step. Physical craving likewise breaks down when nourishment is eaten; emotional appetite, on the other hand, doesn't leave in the wake of eating. It ought to be noticed that yearning signals might be hard to identify after long times of abstaining from excessive food intake and limitation. It very well may be trying to see unobtrusive appetite prompts until they become noteworthy and the individual feels hungry. Working with an enlisted dietitian can be useful in the beginning times of recuperation thus.

It tends to be imperative to find out about what reason this eating conduct serves so the individual can meet their emotional needs more successfully. While eating for solace can be a piece of "typical" eating and is an alternative as aapproach to adapt, it can turn into an issue when it's the main adapting aptitude being utilized. They may profit by working with a specialist to figure out how to be increasingly emphatic, set limits, mend from injury, endure trouble, what's more, other adapting aptitudes to address the hidden issue.

On the off chance that you or somebody you know is battling with enthusiastic eating, ceaseless eating less junk food, or emotional eating, it can be useful to get support from a treatment group. On the off chance that this is causing trouble, it's sufficient motivation to connect. Somebody doesn't have to encounter all indications of an eating issue before finding support.

## Compulsiveeating for women

As a lady, you're most likely acquainted with the urgent drive to eat certain nourishments not long before your month to month time frame. In any case, for what reason is the inclination to eat up chocolate and shoddy nourishment so incredible during that season of the month?

Research shows that premenstrual enthusiastic eating has a physiological segment. As indicated by an examination distributed in the International Journal of Eating Scatters, ovarian hormones seem to assume a significant job. The examination indicated that high progesterone levels during the premenstrual stage may lead to habitual eating and body disappointment. Estrogen, then again, has all the earmarks of being related with an abatement in craving. Estrogen is at its most elevated levels during ovulation.

From a streamlined perspective, you're probably going to feel increasingly disappointed about everything directly before your period. This disappointment might be a trigger for you to eat enthusiastically. Premenstrual gorging ordinarily keeps going a couple of days and finishes once feminine cycle begins, in spite of the fact that this isn't generally the situation. On the off chance that habitual eating proceeds outside of the menstrual cycle, see your human services specialist.

## How might I keep away from urgent eating?

The initial step to decreasing or evading urgent eating is perceiving that the issue exists. You'll additionally need to decide when you're well on the way to gorge. Once you've done this, attempt these tips to help abstain from overeating.

Eat carefully

Keep a nourishment journal to follow all that you eat, particularly on the off chance that you gorge. Perceiving what number of calories you're eating (on paper or through an application) may assist you with halting the cycle. Attempt to eat refreshingly consistently. Cut back on nourishments containing refined sugars.

Burden up on high-fiber nourishments, for example, organic products, vegetables, beans, seeds, furthermore, entire grains. Fiber encourages you feel more full more.

Tidbit savvy

Try not to purchase lousy nourishment. It's harder to eat it in the event that it isn't in the house. Rather, purchase fixings to make sound snacks with an assortment of surfaces and flavors. At the point when the desire to gorge hits, drink a glass of water injected with new natural product or mint. It might be sufficient to check your yearnings. Biting gum or on the other hand eating a candy may likewise help.

For sweet desires, prepare a crisp foods grown from the ground smoothie or a sweet potato bested with a little pat of margarine and a teaspoon of dark colored sugar. Likewise attempt this solid cinnamon maple caramel popcorn formula from Cookie + Kate. In case you're in the temperament for a salty or exquisite treat, make these heated alternative is a blend of curried nuts and natural products, for example, this curried nuts what's more, apricots formula from Family Circle.

Settle on sound way of life decisions

Stress may prompt emotional eating around your period. Working out, rehearsing unwinding strategies, getting ordinary rest, and keeping up an uplifting viewpoint can help oversee pressure. Join a care group, for example, Overeaters Anonymous. Conversing with other people who comprehend what you're experiencing might be useful. You might have the option to execute a portion of their fruitful treatment systems too.

When would it be a good idea for me to call a social insurance proficient? Not every person requires treatment for premenstrual urgent eating. On the off chance that you end up gorging now and again other than the days paving the way to your period, or if urgent eating causes noteworthy weight gain or emotional trouble, you ought to counsel a human services proficient.

As indicated by the Mayo Clinic, treatment for pigging out turmoil incorporates different sorts of mental guiding, for example, psychological conduct treatment (CBT) (CBT) relational psychotherapy (ITP) argumentative conduct treatment (DBT) DBT is a particular sort of CBT with an attention on "feeling guideline" as a methods for checking unsafe standards of conduct. Hunger suppressants or different prescriptions may likewise be utilized. Premenstrual desires are difficult to fight. Furnishing yourself early with information, sound nourishment choices, and stress-the executivesprocedures can assist you with fighting off the inclinations. Know about what you're eating.

# CHAPTER THREE
## *BINGE EATING*

Bulimia nervosa includes visit scenes of binge eating, nearly continuously followed by cleansing and exceptional sentiments of blame or disgrace. Cleansing is a path for bulimics to apply command over their weight or shape. Body concerns unduly impact people's impression of themselves. In spite of the fact that the formal indicative criteria necessitate that binge eating and cleansing happen at any rate two times every week over a time of months, the individuals who take part in these practices less much of the time may likewise need treatment.

There are two types of bulimia. The first is described by binge eating and some type of cleansing. The second is called non-cleansing bulimia nervosa and comprises of scenes of fasting or extreme exercise without cleansing. Binge-eating issue (BED) is unique in relation to bulimia nervosa in that binge eaters don't typically cleanse and they are regularly overweight or on the other hand hefty. Additionally, to get a finding of BED, an individual more likely than not occupied with the conduct for longer than a few months. Similarly as with bulimia nervosa, the individuals who binge less habitually may likewise require treatment.

Be that as it may, binge-eating issue happens all the more every now and again in men than bulimia nervosa, with around two men influenced for each three ladies with the confusion. Both binge-eating issue and bulimia nervosa start during youth or early adulthood. Be that as it may, a large number of the related practices, for example, exorbitantly eating less junk food what's more, utilizing different strategies to control weight, being engrossed with body shape, and at times binge eating or cleansing start prior, now and again in youth. Binge-eating issue is regularly, however not continuously, related with overweight and stoutness. Studies have appeared that as weight expands, the extent of people with binge eating additionally increments.

An ongoing family study recommended that binge eating and stoutness are unmistakable from each other and that binge-eating issue independently expanded the hazard for overweight, especially serious overweight. In this examination a couple of people with and without binge-eating issue, furthermore, more than a thousand of their relatives, were met. For those with a determination of binge-eating issue, some of their family individuals likewise had binge-eating issue. Henceforth, binge-eating issue plainly runs in families.

A few investigations recommend that bulimia nervosa will in general run in families as well. Twin examinations propose that bulimia nervosa is hereditary and inheritable, in spite of the fact that the specific idea of what is acquired stays obscure. Different examinations recommend that people with bulimia may have lower levels of serotonin than individuals without the confusion and that gorging on high-starch nourishments will in general mitigate the condition. Serotonin is a concoction in the cerebrum that manages mind-set, feeling, rest, and hunger. Low serotonin levels may likewise be related with gloom, which every now and again goes with bulimia.

Ecological elements may likewise prompt bulimia and binge eating. The weight on ladies to be flimsy has expanded in the last few years. This gives off an impression of being because of a depiction of ever-more slender perfect body types in the media joined with an ascent in prominence of different sorts of business diet programs. Different components that may add to eating issue incorporate having a family ancestry of weight, being prodded about weight and shape by peers during immaturity, and having low confidence.

Low confidence joined with weight and shape concerns structure the reason for the further improvement of bulimia nervosa and bingeeating jumble. Worry with weight and shape inevitably gives rise to endeavors to control weight and shape by abstaining from excessive food intake. Regularly, such eating less junk food is fruitful in prompting weight reduction yet is in the end followed by loss of power over eating, prompting binge eating.

It begins with my considering the nourishment that I deny myself when I am eating less junk food. This before long changes into a powerful urge to eat. Above all else it is a consolation and a solace to eat, and I feel very high. However, at that point I can't stop, and I binge. I eat also, eat quickly until I am totally full. A while later I feel so regretful and furious with myself.

This book has been composed for any individual who has an issue controlling their eating, whatever their age, whatever their sex, whatever their weight. It is about eating in an uncontrolled manner. It is about binge eating. The term binge used to mean one thing to a great many people: toasting overabundance.

Today the word all the more regularly implies eating to abundance. For some individuals a binge is something flawlessly harmless—a dietary slip or pass, a basic overindulgence. For other people, however, it implies halfway or finish loss of command over eating. This is a significant issue for countless individuals, and not only those in the Western world.

However in spite of the way that binge eating is verifiably boundless, the vast majority know relatively minimal about the issue. Are binges in every case huge? Are they continuously followed by cleansing? Is binge eating a long lasting issue, or would it be able to be survive? Is binge eating a sign that something different isn't right? What kind of individual is inclined to binge and why? How would we recognize—in ourselves or in those we care about—between a genuine binge and straightforward overeating? What's more, most significant of all, in what manner can individuals figure out how to conquer binge eating?

A straightforward method to see this is to consider a binge as the body's method for defeating eating less junk food and keeping up the important caloric parity, in which vitality admission and consumption are equivalent.

A few people experience issues managing pessimistic sentiments or serious feelings of any kind. Rather than taking care of the circumstance that caused these emotions, these people attempt to dodge the sentiments by and large by binge eating.

Breaking the pattern of binge eating and cleansing is amazingly troublesome. The way to recovering power over your eating is to conquered abstaining from excessive food intake.

This can be cultivated first by eating dinners and snacks at standard interims, not more than 2 to 3 hours separated. When eating designs have been standardized, the following stage is to quit limiting your eating routine. One approach to do this is by step by step fusing nourishments you dread furthermore, maintain a strategic distance from into your eating routine. This structures the initial step and is the reason for every single other advance right now. There is acceptable proof supporting the viability of this initial step. In an examination done at Stanford University, people with bulimia nervosa were treated with subjective social treatment.

Binge eating is the utilization of a lot of nourishment in a moderately brief timeframe joined by a sentiment of loss of command over eating. Most people occupied with a binge will quit eating just when they are hindered or when they feel awkwardly full from having eaten excessively. Binges can be huge or little. It is imperative to recognize the two kinds of binges in light of the fact that during treatment huge binges will in general vanish first, littler ones later.

The nourishments devoured in little, or abstract, binges are generally described as "taboo" by the individual and regularly incorporate such things as chocolate, dessert, or cakes. The nourishments devoured in enormous, or objective, binges are generally sweet what's more, high in fat substance. Such nourishments may incorporate frozen yogurt, milk shakes, bread with margarine and jam, cakes, treats, oats, pasta, and so on. Enormous binges don't will in general comprise of dinners (e.g., meat and potatoes).

there is a lot of assortment in binges, albeit every individual may have most loved binge nourishments. There is, be that as it may, another sort of binge eating, known as touching, where people eat limited quantities of nibble nourishments at regular intervals for the duration of the day. At last, these modest quantities mean a lot of nourishment. We have seen a portion of the triggers for binge eating, to be specific, abstaining from excessive food intake, craving, and negative feelings. Different triggers that can add to binge eating when joined with craving and negative emotions may incorporate having a little bit of a "taboo" nourishment, drinking liquor, having a battle with somebody near you, perusing a magazine with include articles on remaining fit as a fiddle, etc. These triggers, joined with eating almost no prior in the day and with constantly eating less junk food, will probably prompt a somewhat huge binge. The prompt triggers for a binge can be very mind boggling, although every one of them are possibly remediable. Despite the fact that binges might be caused by triggers, they additionally, it could be said, serve to trigger various outcomes, including desensitizing the feelings or in any event, annihilating the activating concerns.

## I'm not catching Binge's meaning?

The significance of the word binge has changed throughout the years. It has been in regular use since the mid-nineteenth century when binge implied essentially "a substantial drinking session, consequently a binge," as per the Oxford English Dictionary. While that remaining parts one of its implications, these days word references frequently characterize a binge as far as overeating, and the term guilty pleasure might be utilized. Merriam Webster's Collegiate Dictionary, Eleventh Edition, for instance, says that one which means of the word binge is "an unreasonable and regularly extreme guilty pleasure."

This purported "guilty pleasure" is really a typical marvel detailed by the two people. For some it is an intermittent carelessness, as referenced prior; it has no impact on their lives. For other people, however, for example, the lady whose portrayal opened this part—it is an authentic issue, something that profoundly affects numerous parts of their lives. Inability to get this qualification—among guilty pleasure and binge eating—lies at the core of a lot of the disarray about the conduct.

Perceiving the need to explain the significance of the term binge eating, scientists have explored the encounters of the individuals who binge eat. While no two individual records are indistinguishable, things being what they are, the scenes of eating that individuals see as binges share two center highlights for all intents and purpose: The sum eaten is seen as exorbitant—in spite of the fact that it probably won't appear to be so to the outcast—and, essentially, there is a feeling of loss of control at that point. It is critical to know that specialized meanings of a binge by and large determine an extra element, in particular, that the sum eaten was unquestionably bigger than a great many people would eat under comparable conditions. This size prerequisite is to some degree argumentative, as we will talk about later right now, it is generally utilized.

**The characteristics of a binge**

I haphazardly snatch whatever nourishment I can and drive it into my mouth, at times not in any event, biting it. In any case, I at that point begin feeling remorseful and scared as my stomach starts to throb and my temperature rises. It is just when I feel extremely sick that I quit eating. Individual portrayals of binge eating can be immensely uncovering. What rises is a record that you may perceive on the off chance that you binge or somebody you know binges.

Emotions. The main snapshots of a binge can be pleasurable. The taste and surface of the nourishment may appear to be seriously charming. Such sentiments only occasionally keep going long, in any case. Before long they are supplanted by sentiments of disturb as the individual expends increasingly more nourishment. A few people feel repugnance over what they are doing however by and by keep on eating.

Speed of Eating. Ordinarily individuals eat quickly during a binge. Numerous individuals stuff nourishment into their mouth precisely, scarcely biting it. Some likewise drink bountifully to help wash the nourishment down, which adds to their inclination full and enlarged. Drinking a ton likewise assists individuals with raising the nourishment later on.

Disturbance. A few people pace here and there or meander around during their binges. They may display a demeanor of edginess. They feel the hankering for nourishment as a ground-breaking power that drives them to eat. This is the reason the expression "enthusiastic eating" is some of the time utilized. Acquiring nourishment may take on extraordinary significance; individuals may take nourishment having a place with others, shoplift from stores, or eat disposed of nourishment. Most view such conduct as disgraceful, disturbing, and debasing. I start by having a bowl of oat. I eat it actually rapidly and afterward right away have a few additional dishes. By then I realize that my control is blown and that I will go as far as possible and binge. I despite everything feel extremely tense, and I frantically scan for nourishment. Nowadays this implies going around school searching for nourishment individuals have tossed out. I realize this is truly disturbing. I stuff the nourishment down rapidly. Here and there I go into town, halting at stores en route. I purchase just a little from each store so as not to excite doubt. I stop when I have run out of cash or, all the more as a rule, since I am full to such an extent that I genuinely can't eat any more.

A Feeling of Altered Consciousness. Individuals frequently depict feeling as though they are in a daze during a binge. On the off chance that you have encountered this daze like state, you realize that your conduct appears to be practically programmed, as though it isn't generally you who is eating. Be that as it may, similar to the individual beneath, individuals additionally report that they sit in front of the TV, tune in to noisy music, or participate in some other type of interruption to forestall them from pondering what they are doing.

Everything begins with the manner in which I feel when I wake up. On the off chance that I am troubled or somebody has said something to disturb me, I feel a compelling impulse to eat. At the point when this urge comes, I feel hot and moist. My brain goes clear, and I naturally advance toward nourishment. I eat actually rapidly, as though I'm worried about the possibility that that by eating gradually I will have as well much time to consider what I am doing. I gobble standing up or strolling around. I frequently eat staring at the TV or perusing a magazine. This is all to keep me from speculation, since deduction would mean looking up to what I am doing.

Mystery. A sign of the run of the mill binge is that it happens covertly. A few individuals are so embarrassed about their binge eating that they put forth an admirable attempt to shroud it — and may prevail for a long time. One way they achieve this is by eating in a generally ordinary way when they are with others. Another is by working out significant subterfuge. Maybe you know about a portion of the ways that individuals keep their conduct covered up: for instance, in the wake of eating an ordinary supper, a few individuals later return secretly to eat all the scraps. Others take nourishment to their room or restroom to eat it unafraid of discovery. I go home and go out to shop for nourishment. I start eating before I return home, however it is in mystery with the nourishment covered up in my pockets. When I'm home, appropriate eating starts. I eat until my stomach damages and I can't eat any more. It is just at this point that I wake up from my stupor and consider what I have done.

Loss of Control. As referenced before, the experience of being wild is one of the two center highlights of binge eating. It is the thing that recognizes binge eating from regular overeating. The experience shifts impressively between individuals. Some vibe it some time before they start eating. For other people, it rises bit by bit as they begin to eat. Or then again it might come on out of nowhere as they understand that they have eaten as well much.

Strikingly, a few people who have been binge eating for a long time report that their feeling of being crazy has blurred after some time, maybe in light of the fact that experience has instructed them that their binges are inescapable, so they never again attempt to oppose them. Some even arrangement ahead for what they see as unavoidable binges, in this manner setting up an unavoidable outcome. Preparing permits these individuals to practice some level of authority over when and where their binges occur, in this way limiting their effect. They along these lines feel that they have not lost control. This isn't generally the situation, be that as it may, since they are as yet unfit to forestall the scenes from happening. Besides, huge numbers of these individuals report being incapable to quit eating once they have begun. This is by all accounts the case in any event, when a binge is interfered with—state, the phone may ring or somebody may go to the entryway—as when this occurs, it is regular for the binge to be suspended uniquely to restart once the interference closes.

## How people binge

Individuals fluctuate broadly in how frequently they binge and what nourishments they eat. It is along these lines hard to characterize a regular binge in these terms.

## Recurrence and Duration

To be given an analysis of the eating issue bulimia nervosa or binge eating scatter, two of the three fundamental eating issue perceived in grown-ups, an individual's binges need to happen on normal at any rate once every week. This limit is self-assertive and has changed throughout the years. It has been scrutinized for inferring that individuals who binge less as often as possible, or who do so discontinuously, are less impeded, though this is frequently not the situation. Therefore, clinicians frequently overlook limits of this sort when making a finding. What makes a difference is whether the individual has normal binges and whether their binges are meddling with their physical wellbeing or personal satisfaction.

The importance of the recurrence of binge eating is likewise befuddling. On the off chance that you binge "just a single time in some time," does this mean there is no requirement for concern? At what recurrence is binge eating an issue? Is it the numbers—how regularly you binge, for to what extent, over what time length—that decide how genuine the issue is? Or then again should the managing factor be how a lot of binge eating influences your life? As noted above, by and by clinicians are worried about debilitation—the degree to which binge eating meddles with physical wellbeing or personal satisfaction.

To what extent do binges last? This relies upon an assortment of variables, an especially significant one being whether the individual expects to upchuck a while later.

Information from our patients in Oxford show that, among the individuals who do upchuck, binges keep going on normal about 60 minutes, though among the individuals who don't, they are twice as long. This is very likely in light of the fact that the individuals who regurgitation feel compelled to complete their binge at the earliest opportunity with the goal that they can raise the nourishment and accordingly limit the sum assimilated.

The Foods Eaten in a Binge

The nourishment I eat as a rule comprises of my "illegal" food sources: chocolate, cake, treats, jam, dense milk, grain, and ad libbed sweet nourishment like crude cake blend. Nourishment that is anything but difficult to eat. Nourishment that needn't bother with any arrangement. I never eat these sorts of nourishment typically on the grounds that they are so stuffing. Be that as it may, when I binge I can't get enough of them.

At the point when individuals what binge's identity is asked "What do you eat when you binge?" they commonly give two sorts of answer. The first identifies with the character of the nourishment. So they may answer "sweet nourishment" or "filling nourishment." The subsequent answer identifies with their mentality toward the nourishment. So they may answer "prohibited nourishment," "hazardous nourishment," or "swelling nourishment." What is clear is that most binges are made out of nourishments that the individual is attempting to evade. This is a critical point that we will return to later. It is vital to understanding the reason for some binges, and it is focal to beating binge eating and staying great. You may have perused that binges are portrayed by their high starch content and are driven via "starch longing for"— an across the board legend. Truth be told, the extent of starches in binges isn't especially high, no higher than that in normal dinners. What describes binges isn't their piece in terms of sugars, fats, and proteins, yet rather the general sum eaten. In the event that you binge or know somebody who does, you realize that binges ordinarily incorporate cakes, treats, chocolate, frozen yogurt, etc. In any case, as Timothy Walsh of Columbia University has brought up, while it is generally accepted that these nourishments are high in starches, they are all the more precisely portrayed as sweet nourishments with a high fat substance.

Strikingly, however, the idea of sugar longing for may have had more significance 10 years or so prior. It is my feeling that the structure of binges changes after some time and that it is administered by what nourishments are as of now maintained a strategic distance from or seen as "illegal." Carbohydrates used to be viewed as "terrible" nourishments and in this way included noticeably in binges, though more as of late fats have had the terrible press.

## The Size of Binges

The measure of nourishment eaten during binges differs generally from individual to individual. A few people devour tremendous amounts of nourishment; infrequently an individual portrays eating 15,000 to 20,000 calories one after another. Be that as it may, this isn't ordinary. When individuals are approached to depict precisely what they have eaten and afterward the quantity of calories is determined, a common binge contains somewhere in the range of 1,000 and 2,000 calories. About a fourth of binges contain in excess of 2,000 calories which is near the normal every day calorie needs of numerous ladies.

Research facility examines bolster these records as comparative figures have been gotten when individuals have elected to binge and afterward the exact creation of their binges has been determined. One examination found that one in each five patients with bulimia nervosa had binges of in excess of 5,000 calories what's more, one of every ten had binges of in excess of 6,000 calories. While numerous binges are enormous, it is similarly certain that numerous in any case commonplace binges are little in size in that lone average or even modest quantities of nourishment are devoured. These binges don't meet the specialized meaning of a binge depicted before inferable from their little size, yet the individual perspectives them as binges since the sum eaten is seen as unnecessary and there is a going with feeling of loss of control. The Eating Disorder Examination, a meeting for evaluating the highlights of eating issue that I contrived together with my associate Zafra Cooper, portrays such binges as abstract binges. Conversely, binges in which really huge sums are eaten are alluded to as target binges.

Abstract binges are normal and can be a reason for extensive trouble. They are particularly common of individuals who are endeavoring to cling to aexacting eating regimen, incorporating those with the eating issue anorexia nervosa.

## The Cost of Binges

Spending on nourishment is my greatest single cost each month. Throughout the years it's ventured into the red. Binge eating can be costly and can get individuals into money related troubles. This clarifies to a limited extent why a few people resort to taking nourishment. Scott Crow and partners in Minneapolis as of late considered the fiscal expense of binge eating in an example of individuals with bulimia nervosa. They found that about 33% of individuals' nourishment bills were represented by the nourishment that they expended during their binges.

## Are all binges the same?

Binges shift extensively, from individual to individual as well as inside a solitary person. It is regular for individuals to report that they have more than one kind of binge, albeit a portion of these binges may not fit the specialized meaning (of antarget binge). One individual depicted having three sorts of binge.

## Out and out Binges

I eat and I eat, generally quick, and without pleasure, aside from beginning taste joy which at any rate is tempered with blame. Typically stealthily, and in one place: at home, the kitchen; at school, my room. I eat until I truly can't eat any more. This is normally the sort of binge where I take intestinal medicines—during furthermore, after—which heightens the sentiment of frenzy and blame. Right away a short time later I am so genuinely enlarged that feelings are dulled, yet later I feel horrendous.

## Half-Binges

These generally happen late around evening time and are like out and out binges aside from that I eat nourishment hastily in one spot, and without satisfaction, yet additionally without a lot of frenzy. It is very nearly a programmed response, frequently to some circumstance.

Slow-Motion Binges

Normally I have these at home, not school. I can see them coming ahead of time. I may battle them for some time, yet in the end I yield and have a nearly pleasurable inclination. There's very an arrival of strain at the time since I try not to need to stress any longer. I really appreciate these binges, at any rate to begin with. I pick nourishments that I like and don't for the most part permit myself or permit myself just in constrained amounts. I may invest energy setting up the nourishment. At some stage it hits me what a simpleton I'm being and how a lot of weight I will pick up (not how covetous I am being), and afterward I become significantly progressively blameworthy, however I despite everything feel an impulse to convey on.

Certain gatherings of individuals have unmistakable binges. For instance, individuals with the eating issue anorexia nervosa regularly have little, emotional binges, however these are joined by a similar misery and feeling of loss of control that is related with target binges. Furthermore, the binges of individuals who are fundamentally overweight tend not to be particular as in their start and end can be hard to distinguish. These binges commonly last longer than those of individuals with bulimia nervosa; for sure, they can last practically throughout the day.

## HOW BINGES BEGIN

At this point you might be perplexed by the way that binge eating happens by any stretch of the imagination.

For what reason would something that leaves individuals feeling nauseated and embarrassed happen again and once more? This raises two issues. What causes binge eating issues to start in the in front of the rest of the competition, and what props them up?

Likewise significant, in any case, are the more prompt triggers of person binges. What conditions will in general encourage a binge? Numerous things trigger binges. A great early investigation distinguished the primary triggers of binges and a later one acquired data on precisely where they take place.

Undereating and the Associated Hunger. A few people who binge, particularly those with bulimia nervosa or anorexia nervosa, eat minimal outside their binges. The subsequent hardship can have numerous unfortunate impacts, as it would for any individual who was basically starving oneself. Forcing severe cutoff points on eating and eating too little makes a mounting physiological and mental strain to eat, and once eating begins it very well may be hard to stop. Many state that it resembles a dam blasting.

The inclination to binge typically starts around early afternoon on an "ordinary" day—that is, a day on which I am doing whatever it takes not to eat. During the evening considerations of nourishment become increasingly more of a distraction; and inevitably at around 4:00 P.M. my capacity of fixation will be adequately nonexistent for considerations about nourishment to be thoroughly overpowering. SoI go home and go to the store. One thing that certainly sets me off is hunger. On the off chance that I am ravenous, rather than eating something to fulfill it, I eat anything I can lay my hands on. It's as though I need to fulfill all preferences, in any event, for things I don't care for.

Defying a Dietary Guideline. Numerous individuals who binge likewise diet, and their abstaining from excessive food intake will in general be profoundly trademark in its structure. They are generally attempting to observe severe principles about what, when, and how much they ought to eat. Disrupting such guidelines generally triggers a binge.

Drinking Alcohol. A few people find that drinking liquor makes them powerless against binge. There are various purposes behind this connection. Liquor decreases the capacity to oppose quick wants thus meddles with the capacity to adhere to dietary principles. For instance, an arrangement to eat just a serving of mixed greens could, after a couple of beverages, be promptly surrendered for eating a full dinner. Liquor additionally debilitates judgment what's more, makes individuals think little of how terrible they will feel in the event that they break their rules. Likewise, liquor causes a few people to feel miserable and discouraged, in this way further expanding the danger of binge eating.

Disagreeable Emotions. Unsavory sentiments of different types can trigger binges. Feeling discouraged is an especially ground-breaking boost. Binges start when I'm drained or discouraged or simply irritated. I become tense and panicky and feel vacant. I attempt to shut out the desire to eat, yet it just develops more grounded and more grounded. The best way to discharge these sentiments is to binge. What's more, binge eating numbs sentiments. It annihilates whatever it was that was upsetting me. The difficulty is that it is supplanted with feeling regretful, self-basic, and depleted. Other emotional triggers incorporate pressure, strain, sadness, dejection, fatigue, crabbiness, outrage, and tension.

Unstructured Time. The nonappearance of structure in the day makes a few people inclined to binge, though having a routine might be defensive. Absence of structure may likewise be joined by sentiments of fatigue, one of the mind-sets that tend to trigger binge eating.

Being Alone. As of now referenced, binges for the most part happen stealthily. Being distant from everyone else in this way builds the hazard as there are no social limitations against binge eating.

In the event that the individual is desolate also, the hazard is significantly more prominent. Feeling Fat. Feeling fat is an encounter announced by numerous ladies—it is phenomenal in men—however the force and recurrence of the "feeling" appear to be more noteworthy among the individuals who have an eating issue. In these individuals feeling fat will in general be likened with being fat, whatever the individual's real shape or weight. Furthermore, feeling fat can trigger binge eating.

Putting on Weight. The vast majority who are worried about their weight respond severely to any expansion. A weight gain as meageras 1 pound (0.5 kilograms) may encourage a negative response and, among those inclined to binge, one reaction is to surrender endeavors to control eating with a binge being the outcome. This response depends on a misconception: body weight varies inside the day and from everyday, and transient changes reflect changes in hydration not body fat.

**What Causes Binge Eating Problems?**

**WHY THE QUESTION IS SO DIFFICULT TO ANSWER**

Numerous Processes Are Involved

Mental, social, and physical procedures all appear to have an influence in causing binge eating issues. This recommends ecological procedures assume a job and that these are probably going to be social in nature. In any case, on the grounds that not everybody builds up a binge eating issue, notwithstanding being dependent upon comparative social conditions, extra procedures should likewise be included. Also, as this part appears, hereditarily decided procedures likewise seem to make a commitment, which implies that physical procedures assume a job as well.

Binge Eating Problems Vary in How They Start The examination that has been done on the improvement of binge eating issues proposes that there is more than one course to these issues. Individuals with bulimia nervosa by and large report that their eating issue began at the point when they started abstaining from excessive food intake during their high school years. This may have been incited by a genuine or saw weight issue or by a need to feel "in charge" with regards to challenges throughout their life. Now and again coincidental weight reduction (maybe because of disease) was the trigger. Whatever the precipitant, the outcome is weight reduction, which can be set apart to the point that the individual creates anorexia nervosa.

At that point, after a variable time allotment, authority over eating separates, bingeeating creates, and body weight increments to approach its unique level. A totally different pathway is portrayed by numerous individuals with binge eating clutter. They report a long-standing inclination to indulge, especially when feeling miserable or pushed. This propensity in the long run turns out to be set apart to the point that they create candid scenes of binge eating. In any case, the binge eating tends to be phasic, that is, there are expanded periods liberated from binge eating. This is most dissimilar to bulimia nervosa. To confuse matters further, a few people report a blend of these pathways particularly in the event that they have a blended eating issue.

Binge Eating Problems Vary in Their Course

Binge eating issues fluctuate in their course after some time. For a few, the binge eating issue is brief and doesn't repeat. For other people, repeats and backslides are normal. For others still, when the issue starts it goes on for a considerable length of time. This recommends that extra procedures, frequently separate from those that were liable for the binge eating at the start, become possibly the most important factor to keep the issue going.

As we will find right now part, challenges with connections additionally appear to be significant, as do certain occasions what's more, conditions.

## A CRUCIAL DISTINCTION

When considering the reason for suffering troubles, for example, binge eating issues, it is essential to recognize the procedures that are probably going to have made the issue start in any case from those that lead it to endure. Sothe subject of cause has two sections:

1. For what reason do binge eating issues create?

2. For what reason do they endure?

Two stages in this way should be recognized: the advancement stage (previously the beginning of the issue) and the upkeep stage (after its beginning). Making this qualification not just causes us comprehend the job of all conceivable causes however it additionally has critical viable ramifications. In the event that the objective is the counteraction of binge eating issues, the assignment is to distinguish those procedures that apply their impact before beginning—during the improvement stage—and attempt to prevent them from working. Interestingly, if fruitful treatment is the objective, the errand is to recognize the procedures that are propping the issue up.

## Procedures that contribute to the development of binge eating problems

### Social Processes

As explained earlier, bulimia nervosa seems to have risen during the 1970s furthermore, 1980s in those pieces of the existence where anorexia nervosa was at that point experienced, principally North America, northern Europe, Australia, and New Zealand. Since these are nations where it is in vogue for ladies to be thin, and where eating less junk food among young ladies is normal, social procedures that empower abstaining from excessive food intake may have added to the development of the turmoil. Key among these is the state of style models. Bulimia nervosa developed when being amazingly slight, similar to the English model Twiggy, got elegant. Yet, it isn't improbable that in various societies various procedures may add to the issue. As of late, there has been a transition to counter the effect of underweight style models. In 2006 Spain restricted models with a BMI underneath 18.0 and in the equivalent year Italy required the style business to give clinical evidence that their models didn't have an eating issue. In 2012 Israel restricted models from ads or style appears if their BMI was beneath 18.5; and a comparable line was taken by the style magazine Vogue. Sadly, there are powers working the other way. For instance, a few exercises empower unfortunate weight control rehearses and may therefore advance eating issues.

This is especially valid for those in which a specific (low) weight is required at aexplicit time or where appearance is vital. For what reason should ladies be at more serious hazard? One significant reason is probably going to be the way that eating fewer carbs is a lot more typical among ladies than men and, as we will examine, counting calories incredibly expands the danger of creating eating issues.

This brings up another issue: Why do ladies will in general eating regimen more than men? Two answers ring a bell. Initially, the social weights to be thin are engaged to a great extent on ladies. What's more, second, ladies are increasingly inclined to base their self-esteem on their appearance. Both of these perceptions raise significant more extensive issues concerning contrasts among male and female advancement and the contending and clashing jobs of ladies in Western social orders.

**Ethnic Group and Social Class**

At the point when patients in treatment are considered, bulimia nervosa and anorexia nervosa appear to be to a great extent limited to Caucasian ladies, however tolerant examples are one-sided as for ethnicity. The discoveries of network based investigations propose that binge eating issues are considerably more uniformly scattered. To the extent social class is worried, there is also proof of a social class slant, with patients with bulimia nervosa and anorexia nervosa being disproportionally progressively normal among those with a center or high society foundation. However, this might be because of a predisposition in treatment-chasing with individuals from center and upperclass foundations being bound to enter treatment.

Age, Adolescence, and Puberty

There is solid proof that binge eating issues for the most part create during adolescent years or in early adulthood. This time of beginning can most likely be credited to the way that eating less junk food among ladies is especially regular at this age. The eating less junk food, thusly, is probably going to be the consequence of two powers. In the first place, as of now referenced, ladies are more inclined than men to pass judgment on their self-esteem in wording of their appearance, and this is especially valid right now. Second, at adolescence numerous young ladies start to build up a body shape that goes astray from that thought about in vogue.

This isn't the equivalent for men. In spite of the fact that men are feeling the squeeze to look a certain way, male adolescence makes an appearance that society wants. As young men go through adolescence their musculature and stature increment and their shoulders become more extensive.

Youthfulness itself may likewise be significant. As we as a whole know, this phase throughout everyday life presents major formative difficulties: evolving appearance, variances in state of mind, and changes in social desires and jobs. Youngsters who have the character attributes thought to put individuals in danger of creating binge eating issues—compulsiveness and low confidence—are progressively inclined to encounter a feeling of loss of control as of now. Some find that eating less junk food reestablishes their feeling of being in charge and, as a conduct considered socially alluring by their peers, it additionally gives them a feeling of accomplishment. For them, slimming down might be more about restraint than all else.

The planning of pubertal changes comparable to one's friends may likewise be significant. It is imagined that early improvement in young ladies may increase their danger of emotional challenges since it expands the likelihood that they should stand up to new issues and desires before they are prepared to do as such.

Also, the adjustments fit as a fiddle might be especially hard to adapt to if they happen preceding the remainder of their companion gathering. Specific age-subordinate life changes are additionally important. An especially significant one is venturing out from home to leave to school. It isn't at all exceptional for eating issues to create or intensify right now. It is anything but difficult to perceive any reason why this happens. Not just is the home-to-school progress an unpleasant one, yet for certain young people it is the first occasion when that they have had full authority over what and when they eat. As a result some experience a period of unchecked undereating while others gorge furthermore, put on considerable measures of weight.

**Weight**

Research discoveries show that there is a brought up pace of youth and parental weight among individuals who create bulimia nervosa, and the equivalent gives off an impression of being valid for those with binge eating issue. Normally any propensity to be overweight during the adolescence or young years is probably going to amplify worries about body shape and weight, and along these lines energize abstaining from excessive food intake. Furthermore, having a family part with a critical weight issue may sharpen individuals to "heftiness" and slimming down, causing them to endeavor to stay away from it by confining their eating.

Eating Problems and Disorders inside the Family

It is entrenched that eating issue run in families. The nearby family members of aindividual with an eating issue have an expanded danger of creating one themselves. This could be because of hereditary variables, and the exploration discoveries do for sure recommend that there is a critical hereditary commitment. All things considered, what is acquired isn't known. There are numerous prospects, including the inclination to be a specific weight, natural or mental reactions to slimming down, and certain character attributes. Nor is it clear which explicit qualities are probably going to be included. It isn't far-fetched that "epigenetic" forms contribute; for instance, counting calories may adjust quality articulation.

The way that eating issue run in families doesn't really show that acquired elements are completely or even mostly capable. Conglomeration inside families could be because of natural impacts. Various examinations have been finished concerning the eating propensities and mentalities of the relatives of those with eating issues. To date these investigations have mostly centered around the family members of patients with anorexia nervosa, and their discoveries have shifted incredibly. Some have discovered high paces of surprising eating perspectives and conduct; others have not.

**The theory of binge eating as an addiction**

OA accepts that habitual overeating is a triple ailment: physical, emotional and profound. We view it as a compulsion which, similar to liquor addiction and medication misuse, can be captured yet not restored.

As indicated by the hypothesis that binge eating is a type of compulsion—the alleged "compulsion model" of binge eating—binge eating is the consequence of a basic physiological procedure proportionate to that liable for liquor abuse. Individuals who binge are naturally defenseless against specific nourishments (commonly sugar and starches) what's more, thus become "dependent" to them. These nourishments are "dangerous" to these individuals who, thus, can't control their admission so their utilization logically rises. Since this powerlessness is naturally based, they can never be relieved of the issue (or "sickness"): rather, they need to figure out how to acknowledge it and alter their lives as needs be.

Is the enslavement model substantial? As Terence Wilson of Rutgers University has focused on, these days "the idea of enslavement has been degraded by indiscriminate furthermore, loose use to depict basically any type of redundant conduct." Some of us, we are told, are "sex addicts," others are "television addicts" or "shopaholics."

The outcome is that it is never again clear having a habit. When the word is utilized right now, grasping way, the greater part of us could be said to be "dependent" to who knows what. In any case, there are a few likenesses between binge eating and the work of art addictions including liquor and medication misuse, and numerous individuals center around these similitudes to help the enslavement model of binge eating. They call attention to that regardless of whether the conduct is liquor/sedate maltreatment or binge eating, the individual

• Has desires or inclinations to take part in the conduct.

• Feels lost power over the conduct.

• Is distracted with contemplations about the conduct.

• Might utilize the conduct to alleviate strain and negative sentiments.

• Denies the seriousness of the issue.

• Attempts to keep the issue mystery.

• Persists in the conduct regardless of its antagonistic impacts.

• Often makes rehashed ineffective endeavors to stop.

These similitudes are, be that as it may, halfway. They are fascinating, and some are significant to treatment—for instance, the utilization of the conduct to manage pressure — however the way that things are comparable or share properties for all intents and purpose doesn't make them the equivalent. Also, concentrating only on the likenesses, as it stands frequently done, dismisses significant contrasts between these types of conduct, contrasts that are both vital to the comprehension of them and key to their fruitful treatment.

There are three primary contrasts between binge eating and substance misuse, which are all significant:

1. Binge eating doesn't include the utilization of a specific class of nourishments. Somewhere else Terence Wilson has called attention to that if bulimia nervosa were an enslavement, patients ought to specially devour explicit "addictive" nourishments. This isn't the situation in bulimia nervosa, and the equivalent is valid in binge eating issue. The key eating variation from the norm in binge eating is the measure of nourishment devoured, not what nourishments are eaten.

2. The individuals who binge eat have a drive to evade the conduct. Individuals with binge eating issues, other than those with binge eating issue, are constantly attempting to limit their nourishment consumption, that is, they are endeavoring to abstain from food. What troubles them about their binge eating is that it speaks to an inability to control their eating and conveys the danger of weight gain. There is no marvel proportionate to abstaining from excessive food intake in liquor (or medication) misuse. The individuals who misuse liquor have no characteristic drive to maintain a strategic distance from liquor against the foundation of which their exorbitant drinking happens. Truth be told a significant objective of habit treatment programs is to impart in the junkie the assurance not to participate in the addictive conduct. In most binge eating issues, interestingly, this assurance as of now exists as the powerful urge to control

nourishment consumption. Surely, the drive to control eating is an issue in its own privilege as it propagates the binge eating.

3. The individuals who binge eat dread participating in the conduct. In most binge eating issues, going with the drive to slim down is a lot of mentalities toward shape and weight described by the overevaluation of shape and weight.

Self-esteem is judged only as far as appearance and weight, and these perspectives assume a significant job in propagating the turmoil through empowering tenacious and severe slimming down. Indeed, there is no proportional marvel in liquor or medication misuse. In different words, the craving to confine eating energizes those with binge eating issues to binge. Interestingly, those dependent on liquor or medications are most certainly not helpless against maltreatment of these substances because of their desire to maintain a strategic distance from them.

As can be seen, there are notably various instruments associated with binge eating and substance misuse and these point to two oppositely restricted ways to deal with their treatment. On account of most binge eating issues, treatment needs to concentrate on directing patience. Conversely, medications for fixation need to concentrate on reinforcing it.

Then again, binge eating occurs among certain individuals who don't diet especially seriously, explicitly huge numbers of those with binge eating issue. The binge eating of these individuals isn't driven by eating less junk food, or if nothing else to a far lesser degree. Challenges adapting to pressure appear to be considerably more significant. In this way, conceivably, there is a greater amount of a cover between the components driving their binge eating and those driving liquor or medication misuse.

## The relationship between binge eating and substance abuse

Regardless of whether binge eating isn't itself a fixation, are the likenesses between binge eating and substance misuse demonstrative of a relationship between the two? Could the two issues be brought about by a solitary basic variation from the norm? To answer these questions, considers have been completed to decide how frequently and under what conditions the two issues show up in a similar individual or a similar family.

## Substance Abuse among People with Binge Eating Problems

While advocates of the dependence model of binge eating frequently express that the paces of liquor and medication misuse are lopsidedly high among those with binge eating issues, this isn't the situation. While look into discoveries demonstrate that the rates are in reality raised, they are no higher than those among individuals with other mental issue.

Binge Eating Problems among Those with Substance Abuse

On the off chance that there is a particular relationship between binge eating and substance misuse, those with liquor and illicit drug use ought to have a raised pace of binge eating issues. This does for sure seem, by all accounts, to be the situation, however by and by it appears that is a vague relationship in that there is a raised pace of eating issues among individuals with other mental issue, for instance, uneasiness issue also, wretchedness.

Family Studies

A few investigations have revealed a raised pace of substance maltreatment among the family members of individuals with bulimia nervosa. This finding is fascinating at the same time, similar to the others as of now referenced, hard to decipher. The rates appear to be no higher than those among the family members of individuals with other mental issue. This isn't what might be normal if binge eating issues and substance misuse were the aftereffect of a typical basic procedure.

The Relationship between the Disorders after some time

To comprehend the connection between two issue, it is additionally essential to know whether one will in general lead to the next or the other way around. Investigations of those individuals with liquor issues who likewise have an eating issue propose that the last mentioned grows first. This finding isn't astonishing, in any case, since eating issues regularly start at a previous age than liquor issues.

**The Effects of Treatment**

On the off chance that a solitary variation from the norm underlies both binge eating issues and substance misuse, at that point the effective treatment of one of these issues may be normal to prompt the development of the other (except if the basic variation from the norm had too been adjusted). This marvel is here and there alluded to as manifestation substitution. There is no proof that it happens right now, there is proof that it doesn't, at any rate among individuals with binge eating issues.

# CHAPTER FOUR
## *QUIT FOCUSSING ON WEIGHT LOSS FOCUS ON HEALTH INSTEAD*

I have been battling with my weight for my entire life. I realize I have to shed pounds. I don't care for the manner in which I look. I don't care for the way I feel. I have gone on eats less, attempted industriously to work out, lost the weight, and had everything returned no time. I've lost tally of how often I have experienced this yo-yo pattern of misfortune also, gain. I am completely baffled, embarrassed about myself, on edge also, overpowered about my weight. I am sick of conveying this additional load around. I don't feel better. Consistently is a battle for me. Consistently is a bad dream. I have diabetes now, and I am truly stressed. I dread that I won't be around to see my kids grow up. I am here in light of the fact that I would prefer not to surrender.

There must be an exit from this torment. — Participant in a care retreat

THIS WOMAN IS NOT the only one. Wherever you turn—from TV, magazines, and Sites to papers and radio—you see, read, or hear anecdotes about the U.S. populace's disappointing battle to get in shape. Two out of three grown-ups in the US are overweight, and one out of three is obese,1 more than twofold the pace of corpulence in the late 1970s. Inscientific terms, we are in ancorpulence pandemic, a condition of outrageous weight gain that is surpassing not just the US yet in addition a significant part of the globe. This lofty ascent in heftiness over the past thirty years has no equal in our history, and in the event that we don't change our current patterns, the numbers will keep on rising.

What's more, this is generally in light of the fact that our general public has gotten harmful such that specialists call "obesigenic." We are encompassed by cultural powers that drive us to eat more what's more, move less. Furthermore, the characteristic outcome is weight increase, stoutness, and the bunch wellbeing furthermore, emotional issues that accompany them. Indeed, it's at last an individual choice to eat more than one needs and to not practice enough, but at the same time it's about difficult to get away from the weights around us that lead to undesirable practices. Barraged throughout each and every day by unfortunate outside influences, we handily become separated from what our bodies genuinely require and really need.

Simply think about the nourishment court at the nearby shopping center. It's a gala of decisions that can overpower the faculties. You see and smell nourishments that are exquisite just as those that are sweet—steak sizzling in teriyaki sauce, stove crisp pizza, hot cinnamon buns showered with snow-white icing, rich coffee sugary treats injected with sugar syrup and topped with cream. The plenitude of smells, hues, and sounds stir your sense of taste and your desire to eat. All by itself this isn't really an awful thing—who doesn't cherish the look and smell of delectable nourishment?— yet it regularly prods us to eat naturally whether we're really eager or not. Before we know it, we've eaten a supersized feast that has 66% of the calories we need in one day—and we weren't even ravenous in the first place. At the point when this happens for quite a while, without fail, what started as one agreeable snapshot of eating turns into a weight issue that can affect us the remainder of our lives. Furthermore, this is only one of numerous instances of the effect our environment and interpersonal organizations can have on our weight and wellbeing.

In our nourishment supply, there are a lot of nourishments and beverages that are profoundly prepared with salt, sugar, and fat. As per Dr. David Kessler, previous chief of the U.S. Nourishment and Drug Administration, the nourishment and eatery ventures purposely produce high-salt, high-sugar, and high-fat nourishments just with the goal that individuals can't avoid them and need more. In his book The End of Overeating: Taking Control of the Insatiable American Appetite, refering to look into done in social neuroscience, sustenance, and brain research, he reports that nourishments high in fat, salt, and sugar modify the cerebrum's science, animating the arrival of dopamine, which in turn is related with the sentiment of pleasure. This is one reason that we hunger for a greater amount of nourishments and savors high fat, sugar, and salt—since they are fulfilling.

Promoting is another. It's the market economy's approach to shape social standards that drive utilization and benefits. What's more, with regards to the nourishment business, what they need is for shoppers to really devour—to eat as a lot of nourishment and to drink the same number of drinks as they can stomach, and afterward have some more. It is telling that in the US, the nourishment business spends more on publicizing than some other industry but the auto industry.3 Every day we're presented to many promotions for nourishment and refreshments, every one signaling us to eat and drink. What's more, there is no spot that is off- limits for eating and drinking: we eat and drink in our autos and at our work areas, as we sit in gatherings and as we walk around the shopping centers. It is no big surprise that we regularly second ourselves eating and drinking past what we have to fulfill our actual physiological appetite. We have made a culture of steady nibbling, drinking, and eating.

Presently, think about our social standards around physical action. From the Industrial Upheaval in the mid 1800s up to our present data innovation upset, we have gotten progressively inactive as we depend increasingly more on machines, devices, and autos to accomplish our work and get around. We have definitely lessened the measure of vitality we consume in essence developments what's more, the utilization of our muscles. Also, with the normal home in the United States having more TVs than people, we have become habitually lazy people living under the spell of the TV.

Together, all these cultural powers push us toward eating more calories every day than we use, and without our monitoring it. After some time these additional calories develop, and before we even acknowledge it we've put on a decent arrangement of weight. Also, it doesn't take a lot for this to occur. Throughout one year, one hundred additional calories every day—the likeness eating one little treat or of driving a mile as opposed to strolling it— could wind up pressing ten pounds of additional fat on our bodies.

Given the enormous weight these social influences place on us, how might we get back in contact with our bodies and assuage ourselves of the weight and suffering that emerge from being overweight? In what manner can every one of us arrive at a more beneficial weight? The appropriate response in all likelihood doesn't rest with the present weight reduction industry in the United States. Health improvement plans, diet books, and diet nourishments, herbs, and pills speak to an expected $59-billion industry in the United States. Thousands of faddiet books and weight reduction plans travel every which way. However these almost consistently bomb individuals after some time. You can get in shape on any eating routine, yet there is no scientific proof that inflexible consuming less calories will assist you with accomplishing weight reduction over the long haul.

Despite what might be expected, the U.S. populace is becoming fatter and fatter, and becoming progressively disappointed and disheartened by its inability to get in shape. Millions are spent on innovative work by pharmaceutical organizations to second a corpulence 2x. However, there is still no enchantment pill or recipe that can assist us with losing weight and keep up our shed pounds without side effects. The U.S. Nourishment and Drug Organization is wary in the endorsement of these fat-2ghting medications. However those couple of tranquilizes available that can assist individuals with shedding a couple of pounds have undesirable side effects.

The difficult truth is that the essential law of thermodynamics despite everything holds: When we eat a bigger number of calories than we use, we put on weight. At the point when we consume more vitality through physical action or exercise than we take in from nourishment and beverages, we lose weight. In spite of the fact that this sounds essential and straightforward, the way that such huge numbers of us are overweight focuses to the multifaceted nature of the circumstance. For any individual who has attempted commonly to get in shape, the idea of attempting again may feel like an overpowering and overwhelming errand. Is it really conceivable to change one's propensities for eating and moving, particularly even with a general public that pushes us so hard in the misguided course? How might one start to roll out these improvements?

The Buddha instructs that change requires understanding, and knowledge can't start until we stop and concentrate on what's going on directly before us. This halting, or shamatha, permits us to rest the body and the brain. At the point when we have quieted ourselves, we would then be able to proceed to look profoundly into our present circumstance. We need to step off our rushed life treadmills, to stop unknowingly doing likewise things again and again that have permitted our weight to crawl up. We have to stop, rest, and reflect on a valuable route forward that will end the propensities that have prompted our present weight issues. We should be completely mindful of what is going on in our day by day living. At exactly that point would we be able to start to change.

Changing Your Habit Energy

There is a Zen tale about a man and a horse. The pony is dashing rapidly, and apparently the rider is earnestly heading some place significant. An observer along the street gets out, "Where are you going?" and the rider answers, "I don't know! Ask the pony!" This is additionally our biography. A considerable lot of us are riding a pony, yet we don't have the foggiest idea where we are going, and we can't stop. The pony is our "propensity vitality," the constant power of propensity that pulls us along, that we are regularly ignorant of and feel frail to change. We are continually running. It has become a propensity, the standard of our regular living. We run constantly, in any event, during our rest—the time that we should rest and recover our bodies. We are our most exceedingly terrible foes, in struggle with ourselves, and consequently we can without much of a stretch beginning clash with others.

At the point when a forceful feeling emerges inside us like a tempest, we are in extraordinary strife. We have no harmony. Huge numbers of us attempt to appease the tempest by sitting in front of the TV or eating comfort nourishments. Be that as it may, the tempest doesn't quiet down night-time of viewing. The storm doesn't leave after a sack of chips or a bowl of frozen yogurt. We despise ourselves thereafter for eating the chips and the frozen yogurt. We fear stepping on the scale the following day. We pledge to never do it again. Be that as it may, over and over, we do.

Why? Since our propensity vitality pushes us. How might we stop this condition of disturbance? How might we stop our dread, our gloom, our indignation, and our desires? We need to figure out how to become strong and stable like an oak tree, and not be passed up the emotional tempest. We need to get familiar with the specialty of halting—halting our running so we can be available for and grasp our propensity energies of stress, fault, blame, and dread, and quiet the solid feelings that direct us. We need to figure out how to live completely right now. We need to work on taking in and breathing out with all our mindfulness. We need to figure out how to get careful.

At the point when we are careful, contacting profoundly the present minute, in the present time and place, we acquire seeing, more acknowledgment, more pardoning and love of self also, others; our yearning to mitigate sufferingg develops; and we have more opportunities to contact delight and harmony.

We need the vitality of care to perceive and be available with our propensity vitality so we may keep it from ruling us and stop its regularly ruinous course. Care permits us to recognize our propensity vitality each time it pops up: "Hi, my propensity vitality. I realize you are there." If you just carefully grin to your propensity vitality, it will lose quite a bit of its quality. The chips remain in the organizer, the frozen yogurt in the cooler. The tempest cruises by, and we watch, taking in and breathing out at the same time.

After we become more quiet, we can perceive our weight issue all the more plainly and recognize it as opposed to denying it. This may not be simple for you to do. You may feel irate, baffled, or tired about your weight. Try not to stifle these emotions of outrage. Rather, as the Buddha has shown us, acknowledge and grasp these diHcultemotions, similar to a mother supporting her crying infant. The crying infant needs the mother's caring consideration. Along these lines, your negative feelings and unrest are shouting so anyone can hear, attempting to stand out enough to be noticed. Your negative feelings likewise need your delicate, cherishing care. By grasping your negative sentiments at whatever point they emerge, you can keep yourself from being cleared away by your emotional tempest, and you can quiet yourself. At the point when you are more quiet, you are progressively ready to see that you as of now have inside yourself the force and the apparatuses to start to change.

Halting, quieting, and resting are preconditions for recuperating. On the off chance that we can't stop, we will proceed on the course of decimation brought about by incognizant utilization.

**The Four Noble Truths of Healthy Weight**

The Buddha offered numerous lessons to assist individuals with consummation their suffering, the first and most significant being the Four Noble Truths. The First Noble Truth is that we all have suffering in our lives. None of us can escape from it. The Second Noble Truth is that we can recognize the reasons for our torment. The Third Noble Truth is that we can stop our suffering and that recuperating is conceivable. At last, the Fourth Honorable Truth is that there are ways to liberate us from sufferingg. We can develop our prosperity by solidly applying care to our every day living.

A straightforward model from the field of medication can help represent the Four Noble Certainties. Suppose you are determined to have type 2 diabetes (First Noble Truth), which was likely welcomed on by eating a less than stellar eating routine and getting overweight

(Second Respectable Truth). Your PCP reveals to you the circumstance shouldn't be that way and can be controlled (confirming the Third Noble Truth). You follow the specialist's remedy—taking your medication, eating better, and practicing more—which is your course to mending (Fourth Noble Truth). These lessons of the Buddha begin from when sufferingg was bound to be brought about by an absence of nourishment instead of something over the top, or by a body overburdened with physical work rather than one developed sick from absence of utilization. However they apply to all types of suffering, counting those identified with being overweight.

Presently, how about we reflect upon the Four Noble Truths and how they identify with accomplishing your sound weight. The self-investigation that starts here and proceeds all through this book will assist you with exploring through all the significant factors in your life that affect your weight. It will enable you to find what science-based ways you can follow to arrive at a more advantageous weight. What's more, through your own mindfulness, you can find and choose for yourself what is beneficial and what isn't beneficial for your body and prosperity.

Through the procedure, you will acknowledge whether your weight has affected you genuinely and emotionally. You can turn out to be more in contact with the manner in which you have been eating and drinking, the measure of activity you have been doing or not doing. You can perceive the sum and kind of effort you have been spending to control your weight. You can acknowledge how your work is affecting your day by day way of life and your weight. Through all these reflections, you can pick up experiences from your past that can lead you to progress on your way of mending.

## THE PRACTICE OF MINFUL EATING

To develop care, we can do likewise things we generally do—strolling, sitting, working, eating, etc—with careful mindfulness of what we are doing. At the point when we're eating, we realize that we are eating. At the point when we open aentryway, we realize that we're opening an entryway. Our mind is with our activities.

At the point when you put a bit of natural product into your mouth, all you need is a smidgen of care to know: "I am putting a bit of apple in my mouth." Your psyche shouldn't be elsewhere. In case you're considering work while you bite, that is not eating carefully. At the point when you focus on the apple, that is care.

At that point you can look all the more profoundly and in only aexceptionally brief timeframe you will see the apple seed, the lovely plantation and the sky, the rancher, the picker, etc. A great deal of work is in that apple!

WE HAVE JUST LEARNED that cognizant breathing is a fundamental practice for bringing our body and brain together, sustaining the prosperity of the body and brain, and encouraging our association with all things. What's more, similarly as carefully breathing air continues our physical what's more, otherworldly life, along these lines, as well, does eating nourishment. Not exclusively does nourishment give the supplements and vitality we have to help our physical bodies; careful eating can likewise assist us with contacting the associated nature of all things—and can assist us with completion our trouble with weight.

Taking a gander at the nourishment we eat, we see that it contains the earth, the air, the downpour, the daylight, and the difficult work of ranchers and each one of the individuals who procedure, transport, and sell us the nourishment. At the point when we eat with full mindfulness, we become progressively aware of all thecomponents and e/ort expected to make our dinners a reality, and this in turn cultivates our valuation for the steady help we get from others and from nature. At whatever point we eat or drink, we can lock in every one of our faculties in the eating and drinking experience. Eating and drinking this way, we not just feed our bodies and protect our physical wellbeing yet in addition support our emotions, our psyche, and our cognizance. Furthermore, we can do this various occasions all through the day. Careful eating starts with our decision of what to eat and drink. We need to pick nourishments and beverages that are useful for our wellbeing and useful for the planet, in the humble bits that will assist us with controlling our weight. However there are such a significant number of kinds of nourishments what's more, drinks, thus much data about sustenance thus numerous diet designs, that we can second it very difficult to make the privilege decisions. A decent method to beat this test is to find a workable pace speed on the most recent science-based counsel.

The Basics of Eating Well: What Nutrients Are in Our Food?

Nourishment gives the body the crude materials it needs to run the metabolic procedures of life. All nourishments contain at any rate one, and regularly two or three, of the purported macronutrients—sugars, proteins, and fats. These macronutrients give us vitality to fuel our day by day exercises.

They likewise perform novel jobs all through the body. Sugars give the quickest type of vitality, usable by each cell. Proteins give the structure squares to the entirety of our tissues and organs—skinalso, muscle, bone and blood, liver and heart. They likewise structure innumerable cell instruments and moment errand people, for example, the chemicals that digest our nourishment and the synapses that send signals from the mind all through the body. Fats get woven into the film of each cell, protect nerves, and fill in as an antecedent to life-supporting hormones. Nourishment additionally gives us nutrients and minerals, the alleged micronutrients—truly, supplements that are basic in minor sums—used to assemble tissues and catalyzecompound responses all through the body.

Sustenance study of the mid twentieth century concentrated on understanding what macronutrients and micronutrients we have to kwashiorkor and nutrient D-de2ciency rickets. Beginning in the midtwentieth century, sustenance science moved its concentration to complex interminable illnesses, for example, diabetes, coronary illness, and disease— ailments that grow subtly after some time, have no simple fix, what's more, end lives rashly. On account of numerous advances in science, we presently know a considerable amount about what to eat and drink—and so forth to eat and drink—to forestall these interminable illnesses. However, you don't should be a researcher to eat well. Supplements, all things considered, are found in nourishments. What's more, you need just follow a couple of central nourishment rules to keep up your wellbeing and prosperity. The dietary suggestions that follow are for grown-ups and are adjusted from dietary rules created by specialists in the

Division of Nutrition at the Harvard School of Public Health. Starches, Proteins, and Fats: Choosing the Healthiest Diet books from Atkins to Zone depict starches as the foe. Other sustenance masters tout low-fat, high-starch eats less carbs to get more fit and forestall illness, or push high-protein consumes less calories as the approach to accomplish great wellbeing and a sound weight. Reality with regards to macronutrients and wellbeing, in any case, is that the kind of sugar, protein, and fat we pick is substantially more significant than their relative sums in our eating regimen.

Take sugars. They are found in numerous kinds of entire and handled nourishments—from apples to ziti—yet not all sugars are made equivalent. The most advantageous starches originate from entirety grains, vegetables, vegetables, and entire natural products. The least-solid starches originate from white bread, white rice, pasta and other refined grains, sugary nourishments and beverages, and potatoes. We talk about the purposes behind restricting these less-solid sugars later right now part. Here, how about we center around the positive: Whole grains, vegetables, entire natural products, and vegetables are acceptable decisions as starches, and they are additionally plentiful in nutrients, minerals, and fiber. Entire grain nourishments, for example, entire wheat bread, entire oats, dark colored rice, millet, grain, quinoa, and such—merit extraordinary notice, on the grounds that increasingly more research focuses to the benefits of making entirety grains a day by day propensity. Long haul contemplates have discovered that individuals who by and large, a few servings of entire grain nourishments daily have a 20 to 30 percent lower danger of coronary illness and diabetes, contrasted and individuals who infrequently eat entire grains. Eating entirety grains may likewise o/er some insurance against colon malignant growth, however more research is required on this eating regimen to-illness relationship.

Why Are Whole Grains So Good for Your Health?

Precisely how entire grains ensure against coronary illness and diabetes is still an open research question. What we can be sure of is that entire grains contain fiber, which eases back their processing and makes for a gentler ascent in blood glucose after a feast; the solvent 2ber in entire grains, particularly the sort found in oats, likewise enables lower to low thickness lipoprotein (LDL), the "awful" cholesterol.

The germ in entire grains gives folate and nutrient E, and entire grains are additionally a wellspring of magnesium and selenium—nutrients and minerals that may help secure against diabetes, coronary illness, and a few malignancies. However a few examinations have discovered that the benefits of entire grains go past what can be credited to any individual supplements that they contain.

What appears to be almost certain is that entire grains' wellbeing benefits collect from their extraordinary mix of nutrients.4 The entire is genuinely more noteworthy than the aggregate of its parts—a part of related nature. It's a comparable story with proteins. Plant nourishments or creature food sources can all give the body the protein it needs. Be that as it may, while picking nourishments high in protein, we should focus on different supplements that movement alongside the protein. The most advantageous plant wellsprings of protein—beans, nuts, seeds, entire grains, and nourishments got from them—additionally contain 2ber, nutrients, minerals, and sound fats, and they are earth-accommodating choices, as well. Among the creature wellsprings of protein, some contain restorative fats (fish) or are generally low in hurtful fats (chicken, eggs). But red meat and full-fat dairy items are high in a sort of fat that is terrible for our souls; moreover, as we talk about later right now, red meat, handled meat, and dairy items may expand the danger of a few diseases. Red meat and dairy items additionally cause significant damage on the earth. So to pick the most advantageous wellsprings of protein, both for your own government assistance and for that of the planet, pick plantbased proteins from nuts, vegetables, seeds, and beans. In the event that you do have to expend creature nourishments, pick fish or chicken. On the off chance that you need to eat red meat, it's ideal to restrain yourself to close to on more than one occasion a week. Entire eggs can be a fortifying wellspring of protein yet ought to be expended with some restraint, since eating an egg or progressively a day may increment the danger of diabetes and may expand the danger of heart infection in individuals who have diabetes; on the off chance that you have coronary illness or diabetes, you ought to eat not as much as that sum every week.

Veggie lovers and Protein:

Assortment Is Essential to Good Health

There is one di/erence among plant and creature proteins that is significant for us, and particularly for veggie lovers, to comprehend. Our body takes the protein in plant and creature nourishments and separates it into littler parts, called amino acids, which it at that point uses to manufacture and reestablishtissues and to run a huge number of capacities. Some amino acids are "basic," implying that the body can't cause them and must to acquire them from nourishment.

Others are not basic, and the body can manufacture them by revamping the basic amino acids. Proteins from creature nourishments are classified "finished proteins," implying that they contain all the basic amino acids. Proteins from plant nourishments are classified "fragmented proteins," implying that they tend to be low in at least one fundamental amino acids. All things being equal, plant proteins can meet your day by day protein needs, as long as you pick an assortment of plant nourishments and get enough calories for the duration of the day. Sovegans should take care to eat shifted high-protein veggie lover nourishments consistently—beans (counting tofu), nuts, seeds, and entire grains—to guarantee that they get enough of all the basic amino acids.

The equivalent "quality issues more than amount" message is valid about fats. A few fats are beneficial to such an extent that you can appreciate them consistently, while others are unsafe to such an extent that you ought to harshly constrain them or keep away from them out and out. There is a simple method to tell solid fats from unfortunate fats. The vast majority of the sound fats—the monounsaturated and polyunsaturated fats—originate from plants and are fluid at room temperature. Rich green olive oil, brilliant sunIower oil, the oil that ascents to the highest point of a container of regular nut margarine, and the oils that originate from greasy fish are largely instances of sound unsaturated fats. The undesirable fats—soaked fats—and the exceptionally undesirable fats—trans fats—will in general be strong at room temperature, for example, the fat that marbles a steak or that is found in a stick of spread or margarine. Meat and full-fat dairy items are the greatest wellsprings of soaked fat in the Western eating regimen; tropical palm and coconut oils are additionally high in immersed fat. The trans fat in the Western eating routine comes principally from vegetable oils that have been mostly hydrogenated, a synthetic procedure that makes oils increasingly strong and stable at room temperature—and makes them very unsafe to our wellbeing.

What effect do these different kinds of fats have on our wellbeing?

Various investigations have discovered that when individuals supplant starches in their eating routine with monounsaturated and polyunsaturated fats, their blood-cholesterol profile improves— heart-hurtful LDL cholesterol goes down, and defensive highdensity lipoprotein (HDL) cholesterol goes up. Saturated fats, in the interim, cause both HDL and LDL to rise, so unsaturated fats are a superior decision for heart wellbeing. Trans fats are the most exceedingly awful sort of fat, destructive in even little amounts.8 They drive down defensive HDL what's more, cause an ascent in harming LDL, and they harm the cells that line our supply routes. Research likewise proposes that trans fats trigger inflammation, a red alarm in our invulnerable framework that may underlie various dangerous maladies, including coronary illness, stroke, and perhaps diabetes. Diets high in trans fats may advance weight gain, albeit more research is required into the relationship between trans fats and stoutness. Besides, eating a low-trans-fat diet that is high in sound fats may bring down the danger old enough related macular degeneration.

Trans fats are getting somewhat simpler to stay away from: since word has gotten out about their evil effects—and since producers have been required to show them on their nourishment names in the United States—numerous nourishment producers and cafés have started dispensing with them from their items. It is about difficult to stay away from all soaked fats, in any case, since even energizing wellsprings of unsaturated fats, for example, peanuts and olive oil—contain a modest quantity of immersed fat. So for good wellbeing, appreciate sound fats, limit immersed fat, and maintain a strategic distance from trans fat.

To Control Your Weight, Calories Matter

While there is expanding proof about the best sugar, protein, and fat decisions for wellbeing, there has been progressing banter about the best decisions for weight reduction. Obviously, to get in shape, health food nuts need to eat less calories than they consume. The central issue has been whether the overall measures of starch, protein, what's more, fat in the eating routine hold a specific bit of leeway for calorie control furthermore, weight reduction. A few researchers advocate a low-fat eating routine, while others remain by a lower-starch approach, or a Mediterraneanstyle eating plan, with moderate measures of sound fats and bounty of organic products, vegetables, and fiber. Two very much planned clinical investigations with many members that put these contending diet styles to the test have thought of comparative ends: individuals can lose weight utilizing any of these di/erent systems as long as they lower the measure of calories that they expend; and having social help for making these conduct changes may help them succeed.

So to accomplish a more advantageous weight, the message is to second a lowercalorie eating plan that you can follow—one that allows you to devour sound nourishments that you appreciate—and to second some help for tailing it. A few people may second that help in a formal health improvement plan; some may second it from an online network; some may decide to make thathelp inside their families or friend network, joining or beginning a care living sangha, or by working with associates to get more beneficial nourishments added to the organization cafeteria.

You might be considering what number of calories you ought to expend every day to keep up your weight and the amount to curtail to lose weight. There's nobody answer to that question, since calorie needs fluctuate contingent upon age, sexual orientation, body size, and level of physical movement. A few people may require just 2,000 to 2,500 calories for every day to keep up their weight, and somewhat less to get more fit, while other people who have a bigger body size or are dynamic might be capable to eat more calories yet still get in shape. As individuals get in shape, their day by day calorie needs drop. There are many Web destinations that o/ercalorie-need mini-computers dependent on your present weight and your weight objectives, and counseling a wellbeing proficient, particularly aenrolled dietitian, about your calorie needs is likewise valuable. As a pragmatic guide, a vitality deficit of around 250 to 500 calories for each day can bring about two to four pounds of weight reduction every month, and a protected way to deal with creating this vitality awkwardness is to respectably decrease one's calorie admission and increment one's action. This sums to reducing sugary soft drink by about a can a day and including a lively walk every day.

Eat and Drink for Your Health and Our World: Practical Guides

Past the specialized words like starches, proteins, and fats, there are a couple of down to earth rules to follow that will direct your eating propensities a more beneficial way to control weight and help you bring down your danger of infections.

Go with Plants

A careful eating routine for weight reduction should first and first be a sound eating regimen—both for you and for the planet. Furthermore, the first and most fundamental rule of smart dieting is to move more to a plantbased diet. The wellbeing benefits for eating a plant-based eating regimen are similarly solid.

Many years of research on a huge number of men and ladies has demonstrated that eating an eating regimen wealthy in vegetables, natural products, entirety grains, and solid fats and low in refined grains and undesirable fats can bring down the danger of coronary illness and diabetes. Some examination indeed, even recommends that individuals who eat almost no meat may live more than individuals who follow a more meat-overwhelming diet (in spite of the fact that the science isn't definitive and not all investigations have discovered such a mortality benefit). Veggie lovers and vegetarians will in general weigh less and have lower pulse, lower blood cholesterol, and, thusly, a brought down danger of coronary illness than individuals whose diets incorporate a few or on the other hand a wide range of creature products;20 they may likewise have lower dangers of a few tumors, however the examinations are conIicting and more research is needed. (obviously, for ideal wellbeing, vegetarians must fare thee well to get sufficient nutrient B12, nutrient D, and different supplements they might be absent by keeping away from creature foods.)

There's likewise solid proof of the wellbeing dangers related with eating creature nourishments. The Center for Science in the Public Interest gauges that the soaked fat and cholesterol in red meat, poultry, dairy items, and eggs cause sixty-3,000 heart-diseaserelated passings a year in the United States and another eleven hundred passings per year from nourishment poisoning.23 People who eat meat furthermore, handled meat have a higher danger of diabetes than people who follow a vegan diet. High degrees of red-meat utilization, and any degree of prepared meat utilization, raises the danger of colon cancer, and eating meat, particularly meat that is cooked to a high temperature, may expand the danger of pancreatic cancer. The Nurse's Health Study II, in the interim, followed almost forty thousand ladies for a long time to decide the relationship between red-meat utilization and the danger of getting early bosom disease. It found that for each extra 3.5 ounces of red meat devoured every day—a segment of meat about the size of a medium inexpensive food cheeseburger—the danger of premenopausal bosom malignancy rose by 20 percent.

You don't have to turn into a 100 percent veggie lover to accomplish the wellbeing benefits of a plant-based eating routine. A few examinations have appeared that following a "judicious" diet design—one that is rich in vegetables, natural products, entire grains, and sound fats however includes fish and poultry—instead of a meat-overwhelming eating regimen may bring down the hazard of a few lethal and incapacitating ailments, among them diabetes, heart disease, stroke, and obstructive lung disease, just as bring down the danger of biting the dust from coronary illness, malignant growth, or some other cause. A comparable line of research has discovered proof that following a Mediterranean-style diet design, which is likewise plant based however incorporates dairy and fish, can bring down the danger of heart infection, stroke, Parkinson's and Alzheimer's malady, and disease, as well as the danger of passing on from coronary illness, disease, or some other cause. So you can benefit from turning out to be even low maintenance vegan.

Fill Your Plate with Vegetables of All Different Colors— And Enjoy Your Fruits Whole With regards to vegetables and organic products, the fundamental message comes down to two words: eat more. Individuals who eat slims down rich in vegetables and entire natural products may bring down their circulatory strain too as their danger of coronary illness, stroke, diabetes, and potentially a few cancers. Diets wealthy in vegetables and natural products may bring down your danger of waterfalls and macular degeneration,and therefore help secure your vision as you age.

The benefits of eating entire leafy foods likely collect from the supplements that they give, just as from the nonappearance of less-sound or more fatty nourishments, which they may supplant on your plate. Products of the soil are stacked with nutrients, for example, nutrient C, which gives a lift to the invulnerable framework and furthermore acts as an amazing cancer prevention agent, keeping cell harm from free radicals; nutrient K for solid bones; and beta-carotene, an antecedent advertisement to nutrient An and furthermore a cancer prevention agent. They are plentiful in minerals, counting potassium, which may assist lower with blooding pressure, and magnesium, which may assist control with blooding glucose. They are additionally aincredible wellspring of sound starches, including fiber. Exceptional plant synthetic substances, otherwise called phytochemicals, that give vegetables and natural products their brilliant hues may likewise assume beneficial jobs in securing against malady. Lycopene, for instance, a color that helps make tomatoes and watermelon such a dynamic red, may ensure against prostate malignancy. Lutein and zeaxanthin, different individuals from the carotenoid family, may help forestall age-related macular degeneration.

To get the benefit of all these defensive supplements, make an effort to pick vegetables and natural products in a rainbow of hues each day. Incorporate dim green assortments, for example, broccoli, kale, Brussels grows, what's more, collard greens; yellow-orange, for example, sweet potato and apricots, carrots and melon; red, for example, tomatoes, watermelon, strawberries, and red ringer peppers; white, for example, onions, garlic, what's more, cauliIower; and purple-blue, for example, red cabbage, beets, and blueberries. Make it your objective to expend at any rate five servings of vegetables and organic products daily, since a few investigations second that the hearthealthy benefits of vegetables and natural products start to collect at this level. More is unquestionably better. A serving is about a large portion of a cup of cooked vegetables or cleaved natural product, or one cup of serving of mixed greens.

To make it simpler to measure the part, commit half of your plate to vegetables or organic products at every dinner. Make sure to make the most of your organic product entire, not alcoholic as a major glass of juice. Organic product juice—even 100 percent natural product juice—is high in quickly processed sugar. A glass of squeezed orange has as a lot of sugar and calories as a glass of Coca-Cola. Natural product squeeze additionally does not have the fiber of entire natural product. For sure, the Nurses' Health Study found that ladies who drank a cup or a greater amount of natural product juice every day had a 40 to 50 percent higher danger of diabetes than ladies who drank natural product juice not exactly once per month. Eating entire natural product, in any case, was related with a lower danger of diabetes.

To broaden the benefits of products of the soil past your own wellbeing, purchase your foods grown from the ground from a nearby ranchers' market, or then again purchase an offer in a network upheld ranch. You'll be supporting your neighborhood economy, you'll appreciate products of the soil at the pinnacle of their freshness, and your produce will expend less non-renewable energy sources on its way from the ranch to your plate.

Breaking point Potatoes, Refined Grains, and Sweets

You may see one vegetable that is obviously missing from the rundown of rainbow-shaded vegetables: the potato. While different considers have demonstrated the benefits of eating foods grown from the ground, potatoes don't appear to assume a job in these watched defensive effects. That is on the grounds that potatoes—regardless of whether their skins are dark colored, red, yellow, or purple—share more for all intents and purpose with white bread what's more, white rice than they do with broccoli or chime peppers. Potatoes contain quickly processed starch, and a lot of it.

Eating an enormous part of such dull nourishments can send your blood sugar on an exciting ride. In the first place, as your body rapidly changes over the starch to glucose and assimilates the glucose from the gut, glucose levels rise high; your pancreas siphons out insulin to quickly clear the glucose from the blood, yet it might overshoot things a piece, causing your glucose to plunge a piece lower. This arrangement of occasions may lead you to feel hungry once more, not long subsequent to finishing your feast. After some time, eating abstains from food high in such quickly processed bland nourishments may build your danger of coronary illness and diabetes, and there is proof that constraining these kinds of nourishments in your eating routine may help with weight loss.So eat potatoes sparingly, if by any means, and at the point when you do, don't consider them part of your five-in addition to servings of vegetables daily.

Eating a lot of refined grains and desserts, like eating bunches of potatoes, can cause a quick ascent in glucose, a spike in insulin, and afterward a similarly sharp plunge in blood glucose. Besides, the refined grains that will our grocery store racks—white rice, white bread, white pasta, and anything made with white Iour—are healthfully bankrupt substitutes for entirety grains. The grain-refining process evacuates the wheat and the germ, removing almost the entirety of the fiber and a considerable lot of the beneficial nutrients and minerals. What's left is the dull center, or endosperm. Nourishment makers must, by law, include back some of the lost supplements to refined grains, however they don't supplant everything that has been stripped away.

The American Heart Association (AHA) has suggested that Americans radically cut back on included sugar, to help moderate the stoutness and coronary illness epidemics.The AHA's recommended included sugar limit is close to 100 calories for each day (around 6 teaspoons or 24 grams of sugar) for most ladies and close to 150 calories for each day (around 9 teaspoons or 36 grams of sugar) for most men. Remember, notwithstanding, that your body doesn't have to get any starch from included sugar. A decent general guideline is to skip items that have included sugar at or approach the highest priority on the rundown, or have a few wellsprings of included sugar sprinkled all through the rundown.

Take a Daily Multivitamin with Extra D to Give You a Nutritional Safety Net

On the off chance that you live in the higher scopes, invest a great deal of energy inside, have a brown complexion tone, or are overweight or hefty, you might be deficient in nutrient D without acknowledging it. Veggie lovers and other people who carefully limit their admission of creature items may likewise be deficient in certain supplements, for example, nutrient B12. That is the reason sustenance specialists at the Harvard School of Public Health prescribe that grown-ups accept a day by day multivitamin as "sustenance protection."

There's no compelling reason to purchase an extravagant enhancement. Indeed, even a standard store-brand supplement will have enough of the essential nutrients and minerals that you need. There's additionally no compelling reason to take an enhancement that gives in excess of 100 percent of the day by day estimation of any nutrient or mineral, except for nutrient D, a supplement that is basic for bone wellbeing and that researchers accept may likewise play a job in forestalling constant ailments, for example, coronary illness, a few malignancies, irresistible ailments, and different sclerosis. One billion individuals overall are believed to be deficient in nutrient D, and researchers currently imagine that our day by day nutrient D needs are a lot higher than once thought. Few nourishments are normally plentiful in nutrient D, and indeed, even nourishments that are fortified with nutrient D, (for example, milk in the US) don't give quite a bit of it. Besides, during the winter months, the collections of individuals who live in higher scopes can't make enough nutrient D from introduction to the sun. That is the reason numerous individuals may benefit from taking 1,000 to 2,000 universal units (IUs) of supplemental nutrient D daily. Since a standard multivitamin commonly gives just 400 IUs, you might need to inquire your primary care physician to assess whether you need a nutrient D supplement notwithstanding your multivitamin. At long last, make certain to search for a multivitamin that infers most if not the entirety of its nutrient A from beta-carotene instead of from retinol.

Expending elevated levels of retinol may expand the danger of breaks; pregnant ladies ought to likewise abstain from taking significant levels of retinol, as this may prompt birth defects.

## Breaking point Sodium

Sodium is a basic supplement, yet the vast majority of us get unmistakably a greater amount of it every day than we need. High-sodium diets can fuel high circulatory strain in certain people. Lessening sodium can lower circulatory strain and, over the long haul, can likewise bring down the danger of cardiovascular failure and other heart problems. It's ideal to confine sodium to under 2,300 milligrams for each day—the sum found in about one teaspoon of table salt. Individuals who have hypertension or are in danger of hypertension (counting individuals over the time of forty, African Americans, or individuals who have prehypertension) should curtail further, to close to 1,500 milligrams for each day.

Surely, the AHA presently prescribes that most grown-ups slice back to 1,500 milligrams of sodium for each day, since new research gauges that 70 percent of U.S. grown-ups fall into this high-chance, salt-touchy p g ,group.

One approach to decrease the sodium in your eating routine is to reduce handled nourishments. Nourishment producers add heaps of sodium to solidified dinners, soups, sauces, cheddar, bread, and chips to take into account our taste for saltiness, yet additionally to improve surface and expand timeframe of realistic usability.

Inexpensive food and semi-formal eateries likewise offer particularly salty toll; the Center for Science in the Public Interest, for instance, has discovered that some U.S. café hors d'oeuvres and entrées contain over a day of sodium.

Decreasing handled and eatery nourishments may likewise help you limit the measure of another high-sodium nourishment added substance, the Iavor-upgrading monosodium glutamate (MSG)— and rising look into recommends MSG utilization might be identified with weight. A little investigation in China found that individuals who had the most elevated MSG admission were about multiple times as liable to be overweight as individuals who had the most reduced MSG intake. The findings are fundamental, furthermore, scientists still can't seem to coax out the way that MSG might be identified with weight. It's conceivable that the upgraded Iavor of MSGlaced nourishment spikes individuals to just eat a greater amount of it; it's additionally conceivable that MSG has an e/ect on the cerebrum places or hormones that control hunger.

Get Enough Calcium—But Consider the Source Calcium—the mineral that is basic for solid bones and teeth, the consistent beating of the heart, and endless other substantial capacities — has been the focal point of much scientific banter. The U.S. government suggests that we devour 1,000 milligrams of calcium every day, while the United Kingdom suggests just 700 milligrams every day. A few pundits guess that the U.S. suggestions are molded more by the campaigning of the incredible dairy industry than they are by the logical evidence.

There's additionally been banter about how best to get calcium. The U.S. Division of Health and Human Services and the Department of Farming's Dietary Guidelines for Americans suggests that grown-ups devour three glasses of milk a day. However milk and dairy nourishments are high in undesirable immersed fat. Indeed, even without fat milk has around eighty calories for every glass, and three glasses can truly bust the calorie spending plan of somebody attempting to get more fit.

This discussion over milk gets much progressively convoluted when one thinks about the connection between dairy, calcium, and constant malady. Dairy utilization can secure against colon malignant growth in unobtrusive amounts; elevated levels of dairy consumption all alone, in any case, don't appear to o/er insurance against cracks late in life. If there were no mischief in devouring high measures of dairy furthermore, calcium, this would be simply a scholarly discussion. Be that as it may, examines raise the upsetting chance that elevated levels of milk or calcium admission are related with expanded danger of prostate malignant growth in men furthermore, that significant levels of lactose admission are related with expanded danger of ovarian malignant growth in women.

Also, there is a moral ramifications of drinking milk, since the treatment of bovines on dairy ranches is frequently not exceptionally caring and bovines who can never again deliver milk are then butchered. The dairy and hamburger enterprises are intently connected, so regardless of whether you don't expend the meat of bovines or wear calfskin produced using them, another person does.

So what is the most ideal approach to get calcium? On the off chance that you plan your eating routine cautiously, you can get enough calcium from nondairy sources— among them, verdant green vegetables, calcium-set tofu, and tahini. For certain individuals who eat a veggie lover diet, nonetheless, they may need to consider taking calcium enhancements or making a point to expend calcium-fortified soy, grain, or nut-milk drinks, a little glass of calcium-fortified juice, or calcium-fortified cold grains. On the off chance that you do need to expend dairy items, having a humble sum—no multiple or two servings for every day—and eating a sound eating routine wealthy in vegetables and vegetables can likewise give satisfactory calcium.

An extra benefit of taking calcium supplements is that they are frequently braced with nutrient D, which helps calcium ingestion.

Pick Healthy Drinks

Water is the best beverage decision for wellbeing and weight reduction. Sugary drinks are the most exceedingly awful decision, since devouring them in overabundance adds to the danger of stoutness, diabetes, and potentially even heart disease. Sometimes, in any case, it isn't that undeniable that a refreshment is high in sugar and calories. In the event that you carefully read the nourishment realities mark, you will see that normal "100 percent organic product juice" has the same number of calories and as much sugar as a pop. Grape juice and cranberry juice mixed drinks have more sugar and calories than a pop. In the event that you appreciate juice, stick to one little glass a day, about the size of a good old "juice glass" (4 to 6 ounces). Vitality beverages and sports drinks likewise contain heaps of sugar, however drink advertisers frequently attempt to camouflage these refreshments as "sound" by gloating about the nutrients, electrolytes, cancer prevention agents, or herbs they contain. Try not to be tricked. Remember that there are numerous different kinds of sugar added to drinks— genuine sweetener, nectar, highfructose corn syrup, natural product juice condensed—however to the body, they are altogether wellsprings of additional calories and sugar. Diet drinks, improved with artificial sugars, may not be the best other option, since it is hazy what their long haul impacts are on weight and wellbeing.

The Department of Nutrition at the Harvard School of Public Wellbeing has built up a "traffic-light" framework for positioning drinks. Those most elevated in sugar—

sugary soft drinks, natural product juices, smoothies, and sports drinks—fall into the "red" class: "drink sparingly and in-as often as possible, if by any means." Slightly sweet drinks— those that have close to one gram of sugar for every ounce and are free of artificial sugars—fall into the "yellow" classification: "a better decision, yet don't try too hard." The "green" drinks are your best wager— drinks that are without sugar normally, for example, water or shining water. Tea or co/ee can be a sound decision for most individuals, with some restraint (up to three or four cups per day) and may indeed, even have some medical advantages. Avoid the sugar and cream to keep these refreshments low-calorie and restorative. Pregnant ladies may need to constrain their caffeine. Individuals who get unsteady or have rest issues when they devour caffeine.

## BODY SENSATION AND MINFUL RELATIONSHIP WITH FOOD

Nothing Comes from Nothing

With only a smidgen of care, you can really observe where your bread originates from. It has not originate from nothing. Bread originates from the wheat fields, from difficult work, and from the cook, the provider, and the dealer. However, the bread is more than that. The wheat field needs mists what's more, daylight. So right now bread there is daylight, there is cloud, there is the work of the rancher, the delight of having flour, and the aptitude of the cook and afterward—marvelously!—there is the bread. The entire universe has met up with the goal that this bit of bread can be in your grasp. You don't have to do a great deal of difficult work to get this understanding. You just need to quit letting your mind divert you with stressing, thinking, also, arranging.

Your Body Belongs to the Earth

In current life, individuals will in general think their bodies have a place with them, that they can would anything they like to themselves. Be that as it may, your body isn't just yours. Your body has a place with your progenitors, your folks, and people in the future. It additionally has a place with society and to all the other living creatures. The trees, the mists, the soil, and each living thing realized the nearness of your body. We can eat with care, realizing we are overseers of our bodies, instead of their proprietors.

At the point when we eat we typically think. We can appreciate our eating significantly more on the off chance that we practice not thinking when we eat. We can simply know about the nourishment. Now and again we eat and we're not mindful that we're eating. Our psyche isn't there. When our psyche is absent, we look however we don't it's just plain obvious, we tune in however we don't hear, we eat yet we don't have the foggiest idea about the kind of the nourishment. This is a condition of carelessness, the absence of care.

To be really present we need to stop our reasoning. This is the mystery of accomplishment. At the point when we serve ourselves nourishment and afterward bring it to the table, we don't have to feel we're trusting that others will serve themselves and be situated. We should simply inhale and appreciate sitting. We haven't eaten our feast yet, yet, we would already be able to feel happiness and appreciation. It's an open door for us to be tranquil.

Remaining in line at a market or a café, or trusting that the time will eat, we try not to need to burn through our time. We needn't bother with to "pause" for one second. Rather, we can appreciate taking in and out for our sustenance and mending. We can utilize that opportunity to see that we will before long have the option to have nourishment, and we can be cheerful and thankful during that time. Rather than pausing, we can create delight.

At the point when we can back off and truly make the most of our nourishment, our life takes on an a lot further quality. I love to sit and eat discreetly and appreciate each chomp, mindful of the nearness of my locale, mindful of all the hard and cherishing work that has gone into my nourishment. At the point when I eat right now, not exclusively am I genuinely sustained, I am moreover profoundly fed. The manner in which I eat impacts everything else that I do during the day.

Eating is as significant a period for reflection as sitting or strolling intervention time. It's aopportunity to get the numerous blessings of the Earth that I would not in any case profit by if my mind were somewhere else. Here is a section I like to discuss when I eat: In the component of existence, Webite as musically as we relax. Keeping up the lives of every one of our predecessors,

Opening an upward way for relatives.

We can utilize the hour of eating to support the best things our family members have passed onto us and to transmit what is generally valuable to people in the future.

Focusing to Just Two Things

While we eat, we can attempt to focus on only two things: the nourishment that we're eating what's more, our companions who are lounging around us and eating with us. This is called care of nourishment and care of network. Eating carefully, we become mindful of all the work also, vitality that has gone into bringing the nourishment to us. In the event that we are eating with others, we can see how brilliant it is that during this occasionally rushed life we can discover the time to sit together in a casual manner like this to appreciate a dinner. At the point when you can relax, sit, and eat all together or companions in care, this is called valid network building.

Every Spoonful Contains the Universe

Focus on every spoonful of nourishment. As you bring it up to your mouth, utilize your care to know that this nourishment is the endowment of the entire universe. The Earth and the sky have teamed up to carry this spoonful of nourishment to you. While taking in and out, you just need a second or two to perceive this. We eat in such a way, that each piece of nourishment, each snapshot of eating has care in it. It takes just a couple of moments to see that the nourishment we're holding in our spoon is the endowment of the entirety universe. While we bite, we keep up that mindfulness. At the point when we bite, we realize that the entire universe is there in that chomp of nourishment.

Breathing Comes First

The primary activity when you plunk down with your bowl of nourishment is to stop the reasoning and know about your relaxing. Take in such a way that you are fed. You are sustained by your breathing and you feed other individuals with your act of relaxing. We feed each other.

Killing the TV

In some cases individuals eat while sitting in front of the television. However regardless of whether you turn off the television, the television in your psyche keeps on running. So you need to likewise stop the television in your mind. In the event that there is thinking despite everything going on in your brain, you'll be scattered. To be genuinely present you have to not simply turn off the TV or radio in your home, you need to kill the discussion and pictures in your head.

The amount Is Enough

We don't have to eat a ton to feel supported. At the point when we are completely there and alive for each piece of nourishment, we eat such that each chomp fills us with harmony and bliss. In the event that we are full of this delight, we may find that we normally feel happy with less nourishment.

Setting up a Meal

At the point when you set up a dinner with shrewd mindfulness, it's scrumptious and sound. You have put your care, love, and care into the dinner, at that point individuals will eat your affection. Individuals can completely appreciate the dinner with body and brain, much the same as you appreciate an excellent masterpiece. Eating isn't just supporting for the body, however likewise for the psyche.

The Kitchen

The kitchen can be a reflective practice space on the off chance that we practice careful mindfulness while we are cooking and cleaning there. We can set an aim to execute our undertakings in a loose what's more, tranquil way, following our breathing and keeping our fixation on what we are doing. In the event that we are working with others, we may just need to trade a couple of words about the work close by.

A Kitchen Altar

In your own kitchen, you should make a kitchen special stepped area to remind yourself to rehearse care while cooking. It very well may be only a little rack with enough space for an incense holder and maybe a little bloom container, aexcellent stone, a little image of a predecessor or then again otherworldly instructor, or a statue—whatever is generally important to you. At the point when you come into the kitchen, you can start your work by offering incense and rehearsing careful relaxing, making the kitchen into a contemplation lobby.

Cooking without Rushing

While cooking, permit sufficient opportunity so you don't feel hurried. On the off chance that we know that our bodies furthermore, those of our friends and family rely upon the nourishment we're setting up, this mindfulness will manage us to prepare solid nourishment imbued with our affection furthermore, careful consideration.

Rehearsing Peace while

Slashing Vegetables

Harmony can be rehearsed while cleaving vegetables, cooking, washing dishes, watering the vegetable nursery, and furthermore while driving or then again working. Work on discharging the strain in body and mind and being totally with your task. When you work in the kitchen is additionally the ideal opportunity for contemplation.

Preparing the Table

Eating a dinner in care is a significant practice. We turn off the television, put down our paper, and work together for five or ten minutes, preparing the table and wrapping up whatever should be finished. During these couple of minutes, we can be cheerful. When the nourishment is on the table and everyone is situated, we work on relaxing. "Taking in, I quiet my body. Breathing out, I grin," we rehash three times. We can recuperate ourselves totally after three breaths like this.

Cooking with Joy

Cooking can present to us a great deal of happiness. At the point when I put the water into the bowl for washing the vegetables, I take a gander at the water to see its magnificent nature. I see that the water originates from high in the mountains or from profound inside the Earth directly into our kitchen. I realize that there are places where individuals need to walk a few miles just to convey back a bucket of water on their shoulders. Here, water is accessible at whatever point I turn on the tap. Mindful of the value of clean water, I esteem the water that is accessible to me. I likewise esteem the power that I use to turn on a light or to bubble water. I just should know that there is water and power effectively available to me, also, I can be glad straightaway. At the point when I am stripping vegetables or cooking them, I can do it in care and with affection. I see cooking as an approach to offer sustenance and care to my loved ones. I will handily discover euphoria and harmony in the work. Taking a gander at a tomato, a lot of grapes, or a bit of tofu, I can see the superb idea of these things, how they were supported by the dirt, the sun, the downpour, what's more, the seed. Attempt to sort out your life so that you have sufficient opportunity and vitality to cook in a restful and tranquil way. The vitality of adoration also, congruity in the kitchen will enter into the nourishment that you're cooking to offer to your friends and family and yourself.

A grain of rice Contains the universe

At the point when we take a gander at a grain of rice, one second of care and fixation permits us to see that this grain contains the entire world— the downpour, the cloud, the Earth, time, space, ranchers, everything. Care and fixation bring understanding, and abruptly we can see such a great amount in a grain of rice. It's brisk! Any place there is care and fixation, there is understanding. At the point when you put that grain of rice into your mouth, you are putting the entire universe in your mouth. This is conceivable at the point when you stop your reasoning. At the point when you bite that grain of rice, simply bite, so no reasoning will cut you off from this magnificent reality.

# CHAPTER FIVE
## *DEALING WITH YOUR EMOTIONS*

Have you at any point seen that you regularly don't have the foggiest idea what you feel? Do you some of the time feel like you're strolling around in a passionate mist, realizing that you feel terrible or upset, yet not having the option to truly name the feeling you're feeling? On the off chance that you don't have a clue what feeling you're feeling, it's extremely difficult to do anything about that feeling or to assist yourself with enduring it. When you can put a name on a feeling, you can frequently make sense of some solution for it.

Recorded underneath are four of the primary feelings we experience and some related models. Check whether you can think of different names for every feeling and compose them on the spaces beneath. On the off chance that you make some hard memories concocting various names, recall times when you've had one of these feelings; what did you call it? In the event that you proved unable give it a name at that point, would you be able to consider one for it now? It can likewise help on the off chance that you think of feelings as being on a continuum—as such, there are differing levels or degrees of every feeling. For instance, you probably won't feel precisely furious at your more youthful sibling for needing to go to the shopping center with you, yet you may be bothered or irritated with him. On the off chance that you despite everything experience difficulty, approach somebody you trust for help or utilize the thesaurus on your PC.

The Job of Emotions

Another significant thing to recollect about feelings is that they are there for a reason—they all have occupations. At whatever point you experience a feeling, it's there to reveal to you something. For instance, outrage regularly comes up to inspire us to work toward change when there's something we don't care for about a circumstance; uneasiness comes up when there's something that could be risky to us, spurring us to leave the circumstance or ensure ourselves, etc. Now and then individuals become all the more emotionally delicate, which implies that their feelings get activated more regularly than they have to; you may discover you blow up over something that appears little and wouldn't regularly trouble you, or perhaps you feel on edge in a circumstance where there truly is nothing that is threatening to you. All things considered, you can generally observe why the feeling has come up in you, regardless of whether it is by all accounts an overcompensation. So the fact of the matter isn't to attempt to dispose of your feelings—you need them; rather, you need to have the option to oversee them all the more adequately and not let them control you.

These short stories exhibit how our feelings all have employments. Peruse every storyfurthermore, answer the inquiries that follow.

1. Kayla's folks had separated when she was twelve, and her dad had as of late remarried. Kayla didn't care for the way Mary, his new spouse, treated her— she was frequently reproachful of Kayla, and it appeared as though she was attempting to be Kayla's mother. One day after school, Kayla left her report card on the kitchen table for her dad to see. She was glad for herself for having gotten a B in math, a class she had consistently battled with. Mary took a gander at Kayla's report card before her father could see it and disclosed to Kayla she would need to work much harder, since Bs were not satisfactory.

Circle the feeling that best depicts what Kayla may feel:

Outrage Anxiety Sadness Guilt

What may the activity of this feeling be?

What accommodating move may Kayla make in view of this feeling?

2. Joshua and his better half Emily had been dating for a couple of months. Things had been working out in a good way until the most recent week or something like that, when Joshua began to see that Emily wasn't calling or messaging him as frequently. They didn't find a good pace other much during the week since Joshua made some part-memories work after school and Emily frequently had volleyball training. Joshua had been anticipating investing energy with Emily this end of the week, yet Emily hadn't reacted to his content, and he was

beginning to think about whether she was going to part ways with him.

Circle the feeling that best portrays what Joshua may feel:

Outrage Anxiety Sadness Guilt

What may the activity of this feeling be?

What supportive move may Joshua make as a result of this feeling?

3. Nicole had a contention with her closest companion, Samantha, and they halted conversing with one another. Seven days passed by, Samantha still hadn't called, yet Nicole would not like to be the one to yield. Rather than setting off to the gathering they had intended to go to toward the end of the week, Nicole remained at home and watched motion pictures by herself. She simply didn't want to do anything with any other individual at the present time.

Circle the feeling that best portrays what Nicole may feel:

Outrage Anxiety Sadness Guilt

What may the activity of this feeling be?

What accommodating move may Nicole make as a result of this feeling?

4. Matt had broken time limitation twice a week ago, and now he was grounded. As part of his discipline, his mobile phone had been removed. It was Saturday night and he was exhausted; his folks had gone to visit companions, so he went into their room furthermore, took his mother's mobile phone so he could message a few companions. He nodded off without restoring the telephone, and the following morning his mother inquired as to whether he had seen it. Matt said he hadn't on the grounds that he would not like to stumble into more difficulty and be grounded for considerably more.

Circle the feeling that best portrays what Matt may feel:

Outrage Anxiety Sadness Guilt

What may the activity of this feeling be?

What supportive move may Matt make due to this feeling?

Would you be able to review a period you've encountered every one of these feelings? Take a few time to think about the activity it served and what you did as a result of it, and compose about your encounters in the space gave:

A period I felt irate:

The activity of this feeling:

What supportive activity I took:

A period I felt on edge:

The activity of this feeling:

What supportive move I made:

A period I felt dismal:

The activity of this feeling:

What supportive move I made:

A period I felt remorseful:

The activity of this feeling:

What supportive move I made:

Musings, Emotions, and Behaviors

So far you've been working on naming your feelings and making sense of their purposes. The following significant thing you have to know is the distinction between considerations, feelings, and practices. Regularly we get these three things blended up. For instance, in the event that somebody asks you how you feel, and you react, "I feel like individuals simply don't get me," this isn't really a feeling or feeling, however, an idea. We frequently stir up practices and feelings also; you may think it's bad to blow up, yet what you're most likely considering is the conduct that frequently results from outrage. It's alright to blow up, however it's not alright to holler at others or toss things since you're furious. We will in general stir up how we feel, think, and act principally in light of the fact that these three things are so firmly associated.

This graph shows how our feelings influence our contemplations and practices, our contemplations influence our feelings and practices, and our practices influence our contemplations and feelings. In each circumstance, we experience these three things—we have contemplations about it, we have sentiments about it, and we carry on in a certain way. Add to this the way that each of the three can happen rapidly, and it's no wonder we frequently get them befuddled! To be progressively successful at dealing with your feelings, you have to figure out how to isolate these three things.

For each sentence, circle whether an idea, feeling, or conduct is being portrayed.

1. I detest school. Thought Emotion Behavior

2. I'm stressed over my tests one week from now. Thought Emotion Behavior

3. I can hardly wait to get another MP3 player. Thought Emotion Behavior

4. I get my work done. Thought Emotion Behavior

5. I contend with my folks. Thought Emotion Behavior

6. I'm never going to have a relationship. Thought Emotion Behavior

7. I'm so furious I didn't find a good pace the show. Thought Emotion Behavior

8. I surf the Internet. Thought Emotion Behavior

9. I love my new pooch. Thought Emotion Behavior

10. I prepare to go to the shopping center with companions. Thought Emotion Behavior

11. I don't care for the sweater my grandma got me for my birthday.

Thought Emotion Behavior

12. I'm harmed that my sister wouldn't take me to the motion pictures with her. Thought

Feeling Behavior

Try not to stress on the off chance that you made some hard memories with a portion of these—a great many people are most certainly not used to attempting to think along these lines, so it's normal that it will require some investment for you to become acclimated to isolating your considerations from your feelings and your practices.

Ensure you take a shot at this, however, as it will assist you with having more control over your feelings and the practices that outcome from them. The worksheet on the following page can assist you with sifting through your musings, feelings, furthermore, practices. It's an extraordinary thought to make a few duplicates of it and fill one in at whatever point you're encountering extreme feelings or feeling befuddled about a circumstance; if important, you can return to the worksheet to finish it after the circumstance.

Musings and Feelings Are Not Facts

Because you have an idea or a feeling doesn't mean it's valid. You may think, "I'll never have a closest companion," however that is only an idea, not reality. You might feel disliked, yet that doesn't mean you are disliked—it's exactly how you feel. Our considerations and emotions frequently appear to be consistent with us, so it's essential to recall that they're simply contemplations and emotions, not realities. This care exercise can assist you with working on seeing what's an idea, what's an inclination, and what's a conduct, and that will likewise assist you with withdrawing from your musings and sentiments—at the end of the day, it will help you simply watch your musings and emotions also, recollect that they aren't realities. Until you know about this activity, you may think that its supportive to have somebody read the directions to you.

Watching your considerations and feelings in a waterway

Sitting or resting in a casual position, close your eyes. In your psyche, imagine yourself remaining in a shallow stream. The water comes to simply over your knees, and a delicate current pushes against your legs. As you remain in the waterway, notice your musings and feelings gradually begin to skim down the stream, skimming past you on the current. Try not to attempt to clutch them as they skim by, and don't become involved with them; just watch them as they coast past you down the waterway.

On the off chance that you notice yourself getting made up for lost time contemplating an idea or a feeling so you're going down the waterway with it rather than simply watching it glide past, return to simply remaining in the stream. Take your consideration back to the activity also, center around simply watching. As well as can be expected, don't pass judgment on the musings or sentiments that pass by; simply become mindful of their quality.

Watching your musings and feelings in mists

Here's a second way you can rehearse this activity: Imagine yourself lying in a field of grass, gazing toward the feathery white mists. In each cloud, you can see a thought or an inclination you are encountering; watch each idea or feeling as it gradually skims by. Try not to pass judgment on them, and don't mark them; simply watch them as they coast through your brain. Try not to get the musings or feelings, and don't get made up for lost time contemplating them—simply notice them. In the event that you notice that you've lost it with a specific cloud, take yourself back to lying in the field of grass. In the event that you notice your consideration wandering from the activity, bring your consideration back to watching and marking the musings and feelings, without making a decision about yourself.

Assuming Responsibility for Out-of-Control Emotions

As should be obvious from what you've perused up until this point, feelings are extremely mind boggling. They're comprised of how you feel as well as incorporate physical sensations, contemplations, desires, and practices. The data you found out about your feelings in the last section will assist you with utilizing the aptitudes you'll learn right now section and the by deal with your feelings.

**Three Different Ways of Thinking**

We as a whole have times when we're increasingly constrained by our thinking or rationale, by our feelings, or by a mix of these two; these are the three unique ways we consider things. We should investigate each.

Along these lines of reasoning is what is referred to in DBT as sensible brain (Linehan 1993). Fundamentally, this alludes to the self we use when we're thinking legitimately or genuinely about something. For instance, when you're sitting in math class attempting to work out an issue, you're most likely utilizing your thinking self. On the first day of school, when you're attempting to make sense of where your storage is, you're most likely utilizing your thinking self. At the point when you're thinking from this viewpoint, there for the most part aren't a lot of feelings included; on the off chance that you are feeling feelings, they will in general be genuinely tranquil ones. Check whether you can concoct circumstances when you think from this point of view and keep in touch with them on the lines that follow. In the event that you stall out, approach somebody you trust for help.

Your thinking self is significant, however thinking just from this point of view all the time can prompt issues. For instance, individuals who think from this point of view may consistently disregard how they feel, which can prompt challenges overseeing feelings.

Emotional Self

Something contrary to the thinking self is your emotional self, referred to in DBT as feeling mind (Linehan 1993). At the point when you're thinking from your emotional self, your feelings are extraordinary to the point that they control how you act; you respond from the desires the feelings make in you, as opposed to picking the proper behavior in a circumstance.

Here are a few models: you're feeling extremely furious and lash out at the individuals you care about; you're feeling discouraged, so you shroud away in your room and abstain from conversing with anybody; or you're feeling on edge about a gathering you were intending to go to, so you remain at home. Check whether you can think about a few instances of when you've acted from your emotional self and think of them on the lines that follow. Once more, on the off chance that you stall out, approach somebody you trust for help.

Much the same as with your thinking self, in case you're thinking from your emotional self furthermore, following up on these desires time after time, you'll run into issues. As you can presumably tell from the models over, this is really the self that regularly pushes us into difficulty. So on the off chance that we would prefer not to be acting from our thinking or emotional selves constantly, what would we like to do? The appropriate response is in the third perspective about things—utilizing your insightful self.

Insightful Self

So as to find a workable pace self—referred to in DBT as insightful brain (Linehan 1993)— you have to join your prevailing upon your feelings with the goal that neither method of believing is controlling you and you're ready to consider the outcomes of your activities and therefore act in your own wellbeing. Have you at any point found yourself in a circumstance that may have felt troublesome, however you just recognized what you needed to do? Maybe it wasn't the most effortless activity, or what you truly needed to do in the circumstance, yet it was what felt right, where it counts? That is your insightful self.

We as a whole have this intelligence and we as a whole use it normally, despite the fact that occasionally it probably won't feel like it. Here are a few instances of acting from your insightful self: you blow up with your folks about time limitation, yet you quit contending in light of the fact that you realize they could state you can't go out by any stretch of the imagination; you're at a gathering and somebody offers you medications or liquor, yet you state no in light of the fact that it conflicts with what you have faith in; you have a desire to play hooky however choose to go on the grounds that you would prefer not to get as well a long ways behind. Would you be able to think about certain occasions you've acted from this point of view?

Think of them here, approaching somebody you trust for help in the event that you need it.

For every one of the accompanying stories, check whether you can figure out what direction of believing is being portrayed—thinking self, emotional self, or insightful self—and circle the one that is generally proper.

1. Tanya was at a gathering when a companion passed her a container of lager. She thought, "Every other person is drinking. Will they acknowledge me on the off chance that I don't?" At that point she recalled that she had a significant test on Monday; she acknowledged she wouldn't concentrate well the following day on the off chance that she become inebriated that night, so she stated, "Pass."

2. Ty was extremely anxious about asking Jessica to the prom, however he found a good pace fortitude and asked her in any case. At the point when she turned him down,

he was crushed from the outset, yet then he contemplated internally, "Whatever—it's better along these lines since I can extremely just bear to get one ticket."

3. Makenna was so irate at her folks since they wouldn't release her outdoors with her companions this end of the week. She asked them again close the week's end, yet they weren't moving on their choice. She was so baffled and disappointed that she began to shout at her folks and told them she detested them.

4. Riley frequently stressed over fitting in with different children at school, which made it difficult for him to mingle. One day he concluded enough was enough—he was simply going to begin doing it in any case. He knew he generally made some great memories when he spent time with companions, so he moved toward a gathering of individuals at school and participated in the discussion, despite the fact that he felt restless.

5. Catrina was taking an English test. Despite the fact that she felt it was going genuinely well, she chose to toss in some additional realities, similar to Shakespeare's date and spot of birth, which she figured would get her some extra focuses.

6. Jody was messing about on his skateboard at school when he saw a pack of children watching him. He needed to dazzle them, so he chose to make a decent attempt stunt on the stairs to make himself look great, even in

spite of the fact that he didn't know he'd have the option to land it.

*Since you have a superior comprehension of these three unique methods for contemplating things, it's imperative to begin applying this ability in your own life. The initial step is to survey your examples in the present.*

www.ingramcontent.com/pod-product-compliance
Lightning Source LLC
Chambersburg PA
CBHW070833250726
48662CB00003B/1213